DEPRESSION

Also in the Phoenix Introductions series

Jung: An Introduction
by Ann Casement

DEPRESSION
An Introduction

Barbara Dowds

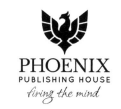

PHOENIX
PUBLISHING HOUSE
firing the mind

First published in 2021 by
Phoenix Publishing House Ltd
62 Bucknell Road
Bicester
Oxfordshire OX26 2DS

British Library Cataloguing in Publication Data

A C.I.P. for this book is available from the British Library

ISBN-13: 978-1-912691-79-1

Typeset by Medlar Publishing Solutions Pvt Ltd, India

www.firingthemind.com

Contents

Part II: Psychotherapy: mobilisation and meaning

Acknowledgements

As always, my deepest thanks go to Peter Labanyi for big and small things: for reading the manuscript and making suggestions, for translating the lines from Rilke, and for all the happiness he has brought me.

I am indebted to the authors of some recent key texts which I have cited copiously: they have saved me a lot of research and reduced my word count as a result of citing them rather than the primary references within their books:

Dana, D. (2018). *The Polyvagal Theory in Therapy*. New York: W. W. Norton.

Dowds, B. (2018). *Depression and the Erosion of the Self in Late Modernity*. London: Routledge.

Gotlib, I. H., & Hammen, C. L. (Eds.) (2014). *Handbook of Depression* (3rd edn). New York: Guilford.

Hammen, C., & Watkins, E. (2018). *Depression* (3rd edn). London: Routledge.

Maletic, V., & Raison, C. (2017). *The New Mind–Body Science of Depression*. New York: W. W. Norton.

Porges, S., & Dana, D. (Eds.) (2018). *Clinical Applications of the Polyvagal Theory*. New York: W. W. Norton.

These books can serve as further reading on the psychology (Gotlib & Hammen; Hammen & Watkins) and biology (Maletic & Raison) of depression, and the application of the polyvagal theory to therapy (Dana; Porges & Dana). My own previous book (Dowds, 2018) explores the interactions between the societal, psychodynamic, existential, and biological dimensions of depression as these manifest in deformations of the contemporary self.

About the author

Barbara Dowds is a humanistic and integrative psychotherapist, supervisor, and trainer, and lives near Dublin. She is author of *Beyond the Frustrated Self* (Karnac, 2014) and *Depression and the Erosion of the Self in Late Modernity* (Routledge, 2018). In a previous life, she was a university lecturer and researcher in molecular biology.

Foreword

The plainness of *Depression: An Introduction* as a title belies the freshness, rigour, and creative synthesis of up-to-date thinking in this book. Both broad and deep in perspective, it offers a succinct examination of the origins of depression as an outcome of genetic and attachment-based developmental patterns in a social, cultural, and economic context. Barbara Dowds does justice to the complexity of depression as a multi-faceted phenomenon and articulates the typical triggers and patterns that occur over the lifespan. This lays the ground for rich clinical illustration of the flexible holistic skills needed to work with anxious and depressed clients.

The book's coherence comes from Dowds' integration of extensive clinical experience and thorough knowledge of current research. The real achievement of the book is to bring so much knowledge into a clear discussion without ever over-simplifying the issues. Social and political change, environmental risks, and even the state of gut flora are linked to the overall model.

Rarely do we read about depression in a way that takes into account and balances childhood origins of depression with triggers in adult life that stretches to include vast social, political, and technological change.

I applaud the urgency, specificity, and prescience of Dowds' reflections on our current political and social climate and its impact on mental health.

Depression: An Introduction is a great primer for students of therapy as well as experienced practitioners who want to grasp how depression is now understood from the consensus of interdisciplinary thinking covering medical, neuroscientific, attachment-based, psychoanalytic, body-centred, and humanistic research and theory.

This is a truly fascinating read and will be of great interest to anyone who really wants to understand what depression is.

Roz Carroll
Co-editor with Jane Ryan of *What is Normal?*
Psychotherapists Explore the Question (Confer, 2020)

Preface

Do we really need another book on depression? I believe there is a place for an introduction that pulls together some of the more specialised work on the topic, presents an overview of the causes, and discusses how practitioners can tackle some of the challenges of treating this most recalcitrant and painful of conditions. Depression is very common and increasing; the scientific basis of our knowledge is constantly expanding; what we think of as a single malady in fact has multiple aetiologies; what are categorised as different psychopathologies are turning out to be genetically related; moreover, depression repeats in episodes which become increasingly resistant to treatment. Finally—and most relevant in a book for psychotherapists—depression is notoriously difficult to work with. While CBT is touted as the treatment of choice and indeed is effective in the short term, its impact is rapidly lost after treatment ceases. This is hardly surprising, since its aim is relief of symptoms rather than tackling the underlying relational and developmental problems. Most of the literature on counselling and psychotherapy for depression comes from a CBT orientation, so there is a case for a broader perspective that engages with both the blocks to treatment and what form longer-term solutions might take.

Chapter 1 contains an overview of evolutionary theories, diagnostic criteria, demographics, and depression through the lifespan. The remainder of Part I examines the causes, course, and consequences of depression in terms of a biological perspective (Chapters 2 and 3); and environmental/developmental contributions (Chapter 4).

Part II focuses on psychotherapeutic approaches. Examined are: what the client can learn from their depression (Chapter 5); blocks to therapeutic engagement and ways of working with such resistance (Chapter 6); psychodynamic/relational approaches for insecure attachment, loss, fragile self, as well as body psychotherapies for working with stress and trauma (Chapter 7); and a case study (Chapter 8). To conclude, there are some Final Thoughts around the theme of hope.

Part I

Incidence, causes, and consequences of depression

Depression is usually characterised as a disorder of low mood, frequently accompanied by other problems such as chronic anxiety. Part I of this book focuses primarily on the causes. The demographics indicate that depression is more prevalent in disempowered groups, whether due to poverty, female gender, vulnerable ages, immigrant status, etc. Such people suffer from lower status and therefore reduced agency in their lives so that they are exposed to far more stress than high status groups.

The specific causes of depression are in part genetic (37 per cent within a population and depending on multiple genes) and in part environmental, most particularly a consequence of stress in early childhood. The genetic component may be important in that it leaves us more vulnerable to adverse experiences in early life, rather than predisposing us to depression *per se*. The reason why vulnerability gene variants have not been eliminated during evolution is thought to be that they provided a selective advantage in surviving experiences—such as abandonment or sickness—that threaten our psychosocial and physiological well-being. It will be argued that low mood is not only a strength under particular environmental conditions, but also that we can learn from the message concealed within the depression.

The development of depression in adolescence or adulthood follows a two-stage trajectory. Susceptibility is laid down during early childhood following a variety of adverse experiences, particularly of the psychosocial variety. Depression may then be triggered in adulthood following stress, bereavement, loss of agency (helplessness), rejection, or abandonment, which mirror the earlier wounds.

Chapter 4 examines the psychodynamic origins of depression, especially as a result of depressed, critical, rejecting, and misattuned mothering. Insecure attachment interacting with other factors such as temperament, genetic vulnerability and life history (e.g. abuse) lays the groundwork for a lifetime of adult depression. We see how depression is associated with deficits in the sense of self and difficulties in relationship. This understanding of the underpinnings of depression leads us into Part II, which details how both client and therapist can work with depression to ameliorate the symptoms and repair some of the developmental deficits that underlie low and stuck mood.

Physical and psychosocial threats, particularly in childhood, leave an imprint on the nervous system; these stress responses are explored in ways that help us to understand not just their role in depression but also how we can work with these patterns in therapy.

CHAPTER 1

An anatomy of depression

Every individual problem is somehow connected with the problem of the age.

—Jung, *Psychological Reflections*

Introduction

Depression is a complex disorder—or set of disorders—often accompanied by (expressed as "co-morbid with" in the psychiatric literature) anxiety or mania. It has been attributed to general childhood adversity, having a depressed mother, stress, inflammation, defective genes, neurotransmitter deficiency, nutritional deficiency, or isolation and existential meaninglessness, depending on whether you are talking to a psychotherapist, psychologist, immunologist, neuroscientist, geneticist, medical practitioner/physician, nutritionist, sociologist, or philosopher. Here I will present a biopsychosocial model, where predisposition to depression is understood as involving both genetic elements and an adverse upbringing which interact with each other, while the social context for parenting may support or undermine child-centred rearing.

Parents' own childhood experiences (e.g. attachment pattern and affect regulation) impact on their capacity to rear their children which, in the absence of intervention, then carries over into subsequent generations: "man hands on misery to man ..."

Evolutionary origins

Bowlby maintained that "Clinical conditions are best understood as disordered versions of what is otherwise a healthy response" (1980, p. 245). Mammals evolved to have emotions which help them to survive and reproduce. Emotions mediate our relationship to our social and material environment; they enable us to adapt by moving towards comfort zones and away from discomfort or danger. Moods last longer than emotions and are less tied to specific cues and are thus an integrated emotional response to our lives that shapes our behaviour (Rottenberg, 2014). That moods offer a selective advantage is revealed in individuals with blunted moods who, it turns out, are less well adapted to challenging environments (Nesse, 2009). Thus, people who don't experience low mood (as in the manic phase of bipolar disorder) generate long-term chaos in their lives, mounting up debts, signing business agreements they cannot begin to fulfil, persuading others they have god-like powers. Likewise, those who have abnormally low levels of anxiety (hypophobia) enter into risky relationships or fail to take safety precautions, get into social or legal trouble, have a shorter lifespan, and can create havoc in society—banks collapsing comes to mind. Mild depression or anxiety carry messages that something is wrong that is demanding attention. Perhaps we are in a relationship where the other consistently puts us down; perhaps our lifestyle is intolerably stressful; perhaps we hold beliefs or expectations (e.g. about success or perfection) that ensure we continually fail to meet unreasonably high goals.

There are a variety of theories for the selective advantage of depression. The social navigation hypothesis suggests it is a way of motivating others to provide help. One theory depends on the observation that low mood is associated with greater realism (depressive realism) (Dowds, 2016). Another argument suggests that because cultural evolution has outstripped biological evolution, our Stone Age nervous systems cannot cope with the stress of rapid change and urban life.

An attachment and separation model holds that the emotions of grief and anxiety keep us close to our attachment partners, while depressive reactions of withdrawal and inactivity give the young animal a better chance of surviving the temporary loss of caregivers (see Dowds, 2018 for references). More all-encompassing views of depression are that it is a reaction to chronic stress or the frustration of our archetypal needs (Dowds, 2018); an effect of processing threats (Gilbert, 2007); or "an adaptation that regulates goal pursuit" (Nesse, 2009, p. 23). The threat to overall fitness (TOF) model (Maletic & Raison, 2017) proposes that the major drivers of depression—social isolation or exclusion and infection—were threats to evolutionary fitness in our ancestral environment (this is discussed further in Chapters 2 and 4).

We can conclude that depression is not a mood *disorder* but an adaptive response to triggers such as loss and stress. Different adverse events lead to a range of—expected—symptoms. Losses are followed by sadness, anhedonia, and appetite loss, whereas chronic stress and failure are associated with fatigue and hypersomnia (Keller et al., 2007). These symptom patterns do not result from stable interpersonal differences, but rather from the specific nature of the adverse events. Thus, "Depression is neither a single condition nor a disease; rather it is a context-dependent and *appropriate* reaction to environmental conditions" (Dowds, 2018, p. 90). Unfortunately, however, depression can then become a learned biological pattern so that later episodes are triggered by less and less stress (a phenomenon known as kindling) as depression becomes a habitual way of being.

Definition and diagnosis

Depression is characterised by low mood such as sadness, numbness, emptiness, a loss of interest or pleasure, and a sense of futility and mean- inglessness. Sometimes the depressed mood is camouflaged by somati- sation or anger and aggression (particularly in men), or by irritability (especially in children), and is frequently accompanied by anxiety and panic attacks. Poor self-esteem with relentless, harsh self-criticism, a belief that everything is fixed ("this is just the way I am") and change is impossible can evolve into despair and suicidal ideation. These affec- tive characteristics are accompanied by cognitive, behavioural, and physical symptoms (Hammen & Watkins, 2018). Depression impairs cognitive functions such as memory, concentration, and decision making, and indeed there can be a significant but temporary drop in IQ during depressive episodes that older people may sometimes mistake for dementia. Behavioural symptoms include either a slowing down or agitation in movement and speech with a withdrawal from social engagement. Depressed people can believe—often correctly—that other people don't want to be around them, but unfortunately the tendency towards self-isolation when taken to extremes only makes the depression worse. Somatic accompaniments to depression include changes in sleep, appetite, and energy as well as a range of other symptoms such as physical pain, fibromyalgia, chronic fatigue, stomach and gut problems, tinnitus, or heart arrhythmia. As for the relationship between affective and physical symptoms: which is the chicken and which the egg? It appears that they are intertwined: physical illness can lead to depression; in other cases, depression can manifest primarily in somatic conditions (Dowds, 2018; Maletic & Raison, 2017). Moreover, compared with people without a family history of major depression, those whose parents suffer from the condition are five times more likely to develop respiratory conditions and a range of other illnesses including cardiovascular complaints, cancer, diabetes, and dementia (Maletic & Raison, 2017).

Psychiatric diagnosis of depression follows either the *Diagnostic and Statistical Manual of Mental Disorders* (*DSM-5*) developed by the American Psychiatric Association (2013) or the ICD-10 depression diagnostic criteria of the World Health Organization (1993). *DSM-5* divides depression into multiple subgroups according to intensity and duration, of which the best known and most researched is major depressive episode, previously called major depressive disorder (MDD). One of the subgroups is bipolar disorder, which involves extreme mood swings between depression and mania, the latter phase being commonly linked with psychotic experiences (delusions and hallucinations). The aetiology of bipolar disorder is thought to be different from unipolar depression, despite the depression having similar triggers and following a similar course in the two cases. This book will be restricted to a discussion of unipolar depression.

According to *DSM-5*, major depressive episode is diagnosed when at least five symptoms that are not attributable to other causes present fairly continuously for at least two weeks, and generate significant distress and impair functioning. At least one of the symptoms is either continuous depressed mood or anhedonia, and the others may be fatigue, hyper- or hyposomnia, increase or decrease in appetite, psychomotor slowness or agitation, very poor self-worth or guilt, poor concentration or indecisiveness, and suicidal ideation. Persistent depressive disorder refers to depressive symptoms that last for at least two years. If the symptoms are mild and chronic, the condition is labelled dysthymia.

Depression may also be categorised according to the triggering event such as winter darkness (seasonal affective disorder) or childbirth (postpartum depression). Having a baby has been shown in some studies to increase the risk of depression, and postpartum depression follows between 7 and 13 per cent of births. The symptoms are those of major depression; and a previous history of depression, poor social support, and stress, including medical complications during pregnancy, all predict postpartum depression (Hammen & Watkins, 2018).

The majority (72 per cent) of cases of depression are accompanied by other disorders, including post-traumatic stress disorder (PTSD), and 60 per cent also manifest anxiety disorders. To a lesser extent (25 to 30 per cent of cases), depression is linked with substance or alcohol abuse. Likewise, depressed people are more likely to suffer from personality disorders, and for those who do, the depression lasts longer. The associated conditions frequently predate the depression, but can occur simultaneously with it (ibid.). When treating any of these conditions, the therapist should be alive to the possibility of co-morbidity and take the combination of disorders into account in the treatment plan.

There have been many criticisms of the *DSM* for being non-scientific, politically influenced, failing to recognise that mental health and illness fall on a continuum, and excluding both the body and the environmental contributions to most or all psychiatric "disorders" and regarding them as emerging solely from brain dysfunction. The National Institute of Mental Health, the major psychiatric research body in the USA, was vocal in its criticism, even before the publication of *DSM-5* in 2013 (Maletic & Raison, 2017). It is calling for diagnoses based on scientific principles rather than the current ragbag of clusters of subjective symptoms, and it no longer funds studies based on *DSM-5* disease categories. As Maletic and Raison (2017) have pointed out, two people need share only a single symptom (e.g. anhedonia) for them to be considered to have the same "disease" of depression. Furthermore, many symptoms such as physical pain and anxiety that are very common in depression have not been included in the "official" list. It matters whether a symptom is considered core to depression or as co-morbid with it because research has tended to rule out participants with co-morbid conditions, thus excluding 72 per cent of the depressed population from studies on depression (ibid.)!

A great deal is now known about both environmental risk factors and a range of reliable but non-specific physical changes in the body and brain that make people depressed. Maletic and Raison (2017) maintain that the lack of a biological marker that is specific to the condition and present in all patients with major depression, as well as the very high frequency of conditions co-morbid with major depression, argue against it as an independent, discrete disease. It is rather a heterogeneous collection of symptoms which are expressions of a spectrum of "underlying pathophysiological disturbances" (ibid, p. 31).

A unified protocol for emotional disorders has been devised that combines anxiety and depression into the single category of "negative emotional disorder" where different kinds or degrees of anxiety and/or depression are viewed as somewhat trivial variations of a shared pathophysiology (Barlow et al., 2011). This way of categorising these types of suffering is less pathologising, and arguably more scientific; for instance, a shared pathophysiology is indicated by the high co-morbidity rates and by the fact that antidepressants function equally well for a wide range of emotional disorders (Johnson, 2019) including anxiety.

Psychotherapy views "symptoms" as defences which were more or less adaptive at the time they developed, but may now be past their use-by date and no longer useful. Thus, the pathologising stance of psychiatry is not helpful to therapists in their client work (although they need to know the *DSM* categories in order to understand the symptoms on which most of the research has been based).

Recurrence and drug treatment

Depression may be chronic (20 to 25 per cent) or occasional, mild or severe, and some individuals may suffer from mild chronic symptoms with episodes of major depression (Hammen & Watkins, 2018). The range of symptoms is similar in the varying degrees of depression, and the different levels of severity seem to have common roots. Indeed, people with mild depression have a five times greater chance of developing major depression, while patients recovering from the worst experience of major depression still continue to have some periods of minor depression (Rottenberg, 2014). Thus, while there are enormous subjective differences between mild and major depression, the risk factors and trajectory are similar, and depression may best be viewed as operating on a continuum of severity.

Those who have one episode of major depression are likely (50 to 85 per cent) to go on to have subsequent episodes, and less and less stress is needed to trigger later attacks (the phenomenon of kindling) so that the probability of recurrence increases by 16 per cent with each episode (Burcusa & Iacono, 2007; Hammen & Watkins, 2018). Conditions that increase the likelihood of recurrence include a more severe first episode, having a co-morbid disorder, or having residual symptoms of depression. Stress predicts first episodes of depression much more than subsequent ones, so different treatments may be called for depending on the stage of the condition.

Virtually all antidepressants since the 1950s are designed to inhibit the metabolism of the neurotransmitters, serotonin and/or norepinephrine. They are partially effective (50 per cent improvement in symptoms) for only 50 per cent of community samples, while "full" remission (more than 75 per cent symptomatic improvement) is only achieved in 30 to 35 per cent of patients (Rush et al., 2006). For patients who fail to respond to two interventions (e.g. SSRI antidepressants and CBT), remission rates with further therapy are no more than 10 to 25 per cent (Warden et al., 2007).

A meta-analysis that included unpublished trial data on selective serotonin reuptake inhibitors (SSRIs) found that patients improved, but no more than those on the placebo (Kirsch et al., 2008). There was a clinically significant difference between drug and placebo only in the case of the most severely depressed patients, and in these instances this was because the placebo worked less well. However, the findings that antidepressants are effective on animals (Keedwell, 2008) is evidence that they have some effect beyond the placebo. Overall, Kirsch's exhaustive analysis reveals that placebos are about 82 per cent as effective as antidepressants.

Other biological treatments for depression are summarised by Hammen and Watkins (2018), but these are constantly being updated.

Frequency, demographics, and gender differences

The prevalence of major depressive disorder (MDD) at any one point in time was found to be 2 to 4 per cent in adults, 6 per cent in adolescents, and less than 1 per cent in children (Kessler et al., 2014) though the prevalence of subsyndromal depressive symptoms is much higher (50 per cent among children and adolescents). These data are worth attention since subsyndromal depression is a powerful predictor of MDD.

WHO World Mental Health surveys (reported in 2011) found a lifetime prevalence of MDD of 15 per cent in ten high-income countries and 11 per cent in eight low- to middle-income countries (Hammen & Watkins, 2018). Lifetime prevalence calculates prevalence to date, whereas some of the survey participants will develop depression in future years. Estimates of lifetime *risk* to age seventy-five were 40 to 170 per cent higher than the lifetime prevalence figures. Depression is now the single largest contribution to non-fatal health loss worldwide, with 4.4 per cent of people suffering depressive disorder and 3.6 per cent anxiety disorders in 2015 (WHO report, 2017).

Depression may be on the increase, one estimate suggesting it doubled in the USA in the decade after the early 1990s. The eighteen- to twenty-nine-year-old cohort was found to have a lifetime frequency greater than the over-sixties, despite having been alive less than a half of the time (Compton et al., 2006). However, Kessler et al. (2014) are critical of this study and cite others which do not demonstrate significant increases in prevalence in the USA and Holland.

Risk factors for depression include female gender, youth, low income (in high-income nations only), lower social class, immigrant status, urban dwelling, illness, or being single or in a poor-quality relationship (Bromet et al., 2011; Dowds, 2018; Hammen & Watkins, 2018). Each of these sub-populations suffers from reduced agency and lower status and is therefore exposed to more stressful life conditions. Since stress is a major trigger for first episodes of depression, it is not surprising that poor women are up to nine times more likely to suffer anxiety and depression than wealthy men (James, 2008).

Gender

Most cultures show a two to one ratio of women to men suffering from depression. The gender difference kicks in during early adolescence and is maintained for the remainder of the lifespan. There are also gender differences in co-morbidity, with women more likely than men to suffer anxiety disorders and men more likely to have a history of alcohol abuse prior to depression (Hilt & Nolen-Hoeksema, 2014). Interestingly, gender differences are smaller in recent than in earlier cohorts, suggesting that increases in gender equality are narrowing the depression differential. The explanation for the gap is probably a complex interaction between psychological, social, and biological factors. Despite a great deal of research, there is poor correlation between mood and hormone levels even though women are most susceptible to depression when their gonadal hormones fluctuate.

Much firmer evidence comes from psychological and social factors (ibid.). Women's much stronger interpersonal orientation causes them to care more what others think of them and to be more emotionally affected by the lives of others. Excessive concern with relationships correlates with depression, and interpersonal stressors more frequently lead to depression in girls than in boys. Prolonged discussion of problems with a friend (co-rumination) improved relationship quality for both boys and girls, but simultaneously led to depressive symptoms in girls only.

The link between stress and depression can be magnified or ameliorated by coping skills (Hammen & Watkins, 2018). In the face of adversity women tend to ruminate (over-analyse their problems) whereas men are more likely to actively attempt to solve the problem or to distract themselves (e.g. through work or sport, but also in dysfunctional ways like drinking). Rumination is not helpful as it leads to self-obsession and intensifies negative thinking.

A much higher proportion of girls than boys are sexually abused in childhood and adolescence (27 vs 5 per cent by age seventeen in the

USA), and female children suffer other forms of maltreatment more than males (ibid.). In addition, girls are more sensitive to certain childhood adversities (parental separation or loss, poverty, discord, and maternal depression) than boys. Women also bear a greater cost in caring for others and suffer chronic strain from unequal power in the workplace and in heterosexual relationships. All of these social and psychological factors correlate with depression and go a long way towards accounting for the gender discrepancy.

It has been suggested that men actually experience depression just as frequently as women, but express it differently through somatisation or externalising symptoms. When anger/aggression, risk-taking, and substance abuse were taken into account the frequency was found to be equal for men and women (Martin et al., 2013).

Non-Western ethnic groups

Comparing rates of depression in different countries and ethnic groups is problematic. The Western concept of the self as an autonomous monad with mind separate from body is foreign to many other cultures, so Western criteria for depression apply poorly to non-Western cultural groups (Eshun & Gurung, 2009). Other ethnic groups may focus on somatic symptoms or on relationships rather than individual emotional suffering. Depression is stigmatised in the Orient, so Japanese (Kitanaka, 2011) and Chinese (Kleinman, 2004) people are more likely to report somatic symptoms such as pain, dizziness, and exhaustion than low mood or thoughts of suicide.

Among US-born ethnic groups, Hispanics and Blacks had lower rates of depression than Whites; and US-born Mexican Americans had a higher risk of mood disorders compared with foreign-born Mexican Americans (Hammen & Watkins, 2018). In the EU, on the other hand, non-EU migrants, particularly first-generation migrants, had higher rates of depression than EU nationals (Levecque & Van Rossem, 2015).

Depression through the lifespan: childhood, adolescence, and old age

First episodes of depression can occasionally occur in childhood, but are much more likely to begin in adolescence or old age, and adolescent-onset depression is more likely to continue into adulthood than the childhood variety (Hammen & Watkins, 2018). The genetic vs environmental contributions may differ depending on the age of onset, the adolescent-onset form being more associated with genetic causes than depression that begins in childhood. Depression that begins in late adulthood is more likely to be linked with neurological disorders than the earlier variants.

Childhood-onset depression

Childhood-onset depression is characterised mainly by somatic symptoms for brief (less than two weeks) but recurrent periods: changes in sleep and activity, decreased pleasure in play, and sadness often expressed as irritability. Childhood depression does not have a genetic component, but appears to have an entirely environmental cause (Rice, 2010). It is strongly predicted by harsh or unsupportive parenting, family stress, and exposure to adverse conditions, including bullying by peers. Depression in childhood is relatively rare, occurring in about 1 per cent of pre-schoolers and 2 to 3 per cent of children under the age of twelve (Gibb, 2014; Hammen & Watkins, 2018). Having preschool depressive symptoms doubled the likelihood of major depression at ages six to twelve. When this older age group was followed up in early adulthood (Luby et al., 2014), most had adverse outcomes, though only one subgroup had unipolar depression. A second subgroup went on to manifest conduct disorder, substance abuse, and social maladjustment, while a third developed bipolar disorder, an outcome that was predicted by a family history of mania.

Vulnerability to depression in children is linked with negative biases in information processing (Gibb, 2014). Like depression-prone adults, they are more likely to attribute negative events to causes that are perceived as internal, stable, and global (the hopelessness model), and they have a tendency to ruminate in a passive and non-productive way about thoughts and feelings (response-styles theory). There is evidence from prospective studies for a role of both of these sets of cognitive biases in predicting and maintaining depression. Specific to children is the finding that their perception of a low level of competence in various domains increases their risk of mood disorders. Children with or at risk of depression also exhibit attentional biases, some studies showing preferential attention to sad faces, and others avoiding these stimuli. Finally, depressed children have personal memory biases with fewer specific autobiographical memories than either control groups or children with other kinds of psychopathology. Whether the overgeneralised memory is a cause, consequence, or simply a correlate of depression is not yet known, but it is notable that the lack of emotionally suffused detail occurs also in individuals with the avoidant kind of insecure attachment (Chapter 4).

Adolescent-onset depression

Depression in adolescence is associated with higher rates of social difficulties, academic failure, teenage pregnancy, partner violence, health problems, and suicidal behaviour. The period from adolescence through the mid-twenties is now one of the most common periods for the first appearance of major depression, and unfortunately depression in adolescence predicts depression in adulthood (Rudolph & Flynn, 2014). By mid- to late adolescence, rates of clinical depression are similar to adult rates (15 to 25 per cent prevalence), but a much greater proportion (20 to 50 per cent) suffer significant depressive symptoms. Teenage depression is associated with anxiety and conduct disorders, and indeed there is a shared genetic liability for these three supposedly separate conditions.

Male and female rates of depression begin to diverge at the age of thirteen and reach the adult ratio of two to one females to males by the age of eighteen (Gibb, 2014). There is very inconsistent evidence for the hypothesis that hormonal changes play a direct role in the gender divergence (Hilt & Nolen-Hoeksema, 2014). However, one risk factor for depression in girls is early onset of puberty (or even perceived early timing—Rudolph & Flynn, 2014). This could be partly because there is a correlation between early puberty and an adverse environment (harsh parenting, poverty, and family instability), but equally may arise from the meanings attributed to maturation. These can differ markedly between boys and girls, with girls more likely to reject the body changes, particularly weight gain, that puberty can bring. Unfortunately, societal mores do not help them, since fashion in developed nations favours the prepubescent look.

A difficulty for both genders in adolescence arises from the disjunction between physical and mental maturation. In adolescence the parts of the brain that regulate judgement and executive functions mature later than those that control emotional reactivity, arousal, and motivation. The dysregulation has different outcomes for boys and girls, with girls more likely to develop internalising disorders and boys externalising ones. Such emotional dysregulation is exacerbated by early hormonal development because early-onset puberty is linked with early sexual relationships at an age where the young girl is less able to process concerns about body image, relationship instability and conflict, sexual rejection, and other wounds to self-esteem and attachment security (Hammen & Watkins, 2018). Hormonal maturation rather than age predicts greater reactivity to unambiguous social threat (Rudolph & Flynn, 2014).

Age of menarche is not just phenotypically linked to depression (above), but there is also a small genetic/causal correlation (r = –0.12) via a gene involved in regulating cell pluripotency and the inflammatory response. There is additionally a small genetic correlation between age of menopause and depression (r = –0.11) (see Howard et al., 2019 and references therein). Thus, there may be a small genetic contribution shared between earlier female reproductive transitions and depression.

Both clinical and subclinical levels of depressive symptoms in adolescence predict elevated rates of major depression in adulthood, with 25 to 45 per cent recurrence over various periods of time (references in Hammen & Watkins, 2018, p. 45). Because adolescence is such a crucial and wide-ranging period of development (establishing autonomy, the formation of peer relationships, learning all sorts of skills for independent living, and acquiring an education and paid work), it is particularly important to intervene in depression that begins during the teenage years and early twenties.

The heritability for depression in adulthood is under 40 per cent, and this genetic contribution is activated in adolescence, particularly in girls. Genetic vulnerability along with early social adversity combine to make some young people more sensitive than others to the trials of adolescence. Parenting in both childhood and the teenage years contributes to maladaptive patterns: for example, emotional competence may not be developed; positive emotions may not be reinforced while negative are; and parents may model or teach disengagement from stress rather than learning effective responses to it (Rudolph & Flynn, 2014). These risk factors combine to produce cognitive, emotional, and relational outcomes that increase susceptibility to the stress of the adolescent transition—of which social stress forms the greatest part (ibid.). Cognitive attributes include rigid thinking; depressive inferences and attributions; attentional and memory biases; and a tendency to ruminate.

Difficulties with processing and regulating emotions are core to depression. These patterns include trait-like higher levels of negative and lower levels of positive emotionality; reduced reward expectation following positive outcomes; more avoidance of and less engagement with goals and plans. Individuals with depression exhibit maladaptive behaviours that elicit negative interpersonal reactions. For example, they may feel little trust in the other; are often exceptionally sensitive to perceived slights; and appraise themselves in a negative way. This lack of confidence in their capacity to fit in socially then results in an excessive negative focus on the self, and constant seeking of reassurance. The outcome can be self-isolation, mixing only with other marginalised young people, or suffering outright rejection by peers. These emotional, interpersonal, and cognitive patterns all heighten reactivity to a stage in life that is already full of stressful challenges as adolescents make the transition to the society of their peers and entry into adult independence.

A birth cohort effect of high rates of depression in adolescence began in the late twentieth century and is found throughout the developed world. In contrast to people born in the first half of the century, those born since 1955 display the highest rates of major depression by age twenty-five, and youth suicide rates increased dramatically until 1990 in the USA. The breakdown in both family and community stability are possible reasons for this, alongside greater pressures to find meaning through individual success rather than shared ideals or goals, or religious beliefs (Hammen & Watkins, 2018).

Late-life depression

The WHO report of 2017 estimated that depression rates peaked in older adulthood (age fifty-five to seventy-four) when 7.5 per cent of women and 5.5 per cent of men were found to suffer from this condition worldwide. Half of cases of late-life depression are thought to be first onsets.

The rates in old age (over sixty-fives) depend on the population sample, being lower than among younger people in high-income nations, but higher in low- to middle-income countries. Both major and minor depression are more prevalent in clinical than community samples, the combined prevalence being 11 to 23 per cent among hospitalised patients, and 12 per cent (MDD) and 30 per cent (minor depression) for institutionalised older adults. Different results are obtained depending on the assessment method: depressive symptom scores increased linearly after the age of sixty-five in correlation with the onset of other medical problems, whereas diagnoses of clinical depression decreased at sixty-five, but increased again after the age of eighty-five. Rates of suicide used to be highest among the elderly in the USA, but they have declined between 1991 and 2009, and have been lower in the over sixty-fives compared with the twenty-five to sixty-four age group since 2005 (Blazer & Hybels, 2014).

Only a small amount of the variance for depression in older adults is caused by genetic contributions—16 to 19 per cent depending on the symptoms, according to a Swedish study, compared to 37 per cent in adulthood overall. Late life depression is higher in people with personality disorders as well as among those who score high on the personality trait of neuroticism (one of the five OCEAN personality traits).

As with other age groups, older people responded to adverse events with greater negativity or cognitive distortion. However, the elderly overall are more likely to attend to and remember positive experiences compared to younger adults. Likewise, the wisdom of age reduces the risk of depression. Social risk factors for late-onset depression include bereavement, loneliness, and life-threatening illness. But other adverse events such as divorce or trouble with the law are less common in later life.

Despite such protective elements, depression is the most common type of emotional suffering in later life and the form it takes at this stage can be somewhat different from earlier onsets. Old people are less likely to combine depression with anxiety, and triggering events are commonly different from early-onset depression. Depression is often linked with cognitive impairment in later life, and this is reversible when the depression improves, unless there are other medical problems with overlapping symptoms. However, the depression of late life can be difficult to distinguish from conditions such as vascular dementia, stroke, Alzheimer's and Parkinson's diseases, or simply the declines in energy, mobility, appetite, and sleep that are part and parcel of the ageing process. Other chronic medical illnesses that are linked with depression include cardiovascular disease and diabetes. Depression can cause medical problems, and medical problems can lead to depression, so the causation is bidirectional (Blazer & Hybels, 2014).

Sadness and loneliness in late life can be ameliorated and prevented from turning into major depression by enhancing self-efficacy. This may involve improving physical health and physical performance, enhancing cognitive functioning, developing greater coping strategies, and improving social skills. Depression is chronic and recurrent, and the prognosis is similar for older and younger adults in cases where the former group does not suffer medical illness, or physical or cognitive impairment. However, poor social support and physical limitations both predict poor outcomes.

Conclusions

Depression is a heterogeneous collection of interconnected conditions. In most cases, it is accompanied by other mood, conduct, or personality disorders: for example, 60 per cent of depressed clients also suffer from anxiety disorders, and about 30 per cent show substance or alcohol abuse, which may predate the depression or constitute an attempt to self-medicate the low or anxious mood. Because of this, treatment should aim to tackle the underlying cause (such as adverse childhood and/or trauma) as well as to ameliorate a wide range of symptoms. Depression is not only characterised by anhedonia and poor self-esteem, but also tends to embrace a variety of somatic symptoms such as dysregulated sleep, eating and energy patterns, pain, and digestive difficulties, and it carries an increased risk of developing a range of physical illnesses.

Depression is triggered by stress, but it is chronic and recurrent, and less stress is needed to provoke later episodes (kindling). Risk factors for depression include adverse conditions in childhood, having reduced agency and lower status (including female gender and lower social class) in adulthood, as well as genetic vulnerability which interacts with the environmental triggers. It is axiomatic that being relatively powerless exposes an individual to greater stress and poor self-esteem.

First episodes can occur in childhood, but depression is far more likely to begin in adolescence or old age. The genetic contribution peaks at 37 per cent in the depression of adolescence and young adulthood, whereas it is a smaller component in late-life onset and plays no role in childhood depression, which is entirely caused by adverse experiences. Late-life onset can easily be confused with neurodegenerative conditions such as dementia, so it is important to ask for a thorough medical check first when working with older clients. Rates of clinical depression in adolescence are similar to rates in adulthood, but a larger proportion of adolescents also suffer subclinical symptoms. Female and male rates of depression begin to diverge at puberty, until they reach the two to one ratio observed worldwide in adulthood. It is crucial to intervene and treat depression that arises in adolescence, not only because this is such an important developmental phase for transitioning into adulthood, but also in order to pre-empt the kindling effect. In the absence of early intervention, the individual faces a life punctuated by depressive episodes, with each attack generating increased vulnerability to further episodes.

Depression is an extreme version of a healthy response: it has not been eliminated by natural selection because low mood helps us to survive a variety of threats to our emotional, social, and physiological well-being. A key process in psychotherapy is searching for the message hidden within the low mood. The therapist must ask how the clients' priorities, beliefs, values, and way of life no longer serve them, and help them to become more empowered, and to build up the social support on which we all depend. If a first episode of depression is seen as a wake-up call rather than a disease, the individual can learn and profit from it.

CHAPTER 2

Biological causes and consequences

In this chapter we explore the interactive roles of genetic make-up and the rearing environment on liability to depression as well as the mechanisms whereby this disorder can be passed on intergenerationally. We will examine how changes in the immune system, the stress responses, and the digestive system can serve as both causes and consequences of depression.

Evolution of depression

A significant part (37 per cent) of our vulnerability to depression can be attributed to our genetic make-up, which raises the question as to why genetic variants that contribute to such a crippling disability were not culled by natural selection. There are two sets of theories: one, that these mutations are damaging but haven't yet been selected out; and the second that they are in fact beneficial. Nonadaptive hypotheses suggest that because of its polygenic nature, alleles contributing to depression are collectively common, but individually recent and rare and therefore have yet to be eliminated by natural selection despite being maladaptive (Maletic & Raison, 2017). Adaptive theories, on the other hand, propose that symptoms of depression actually benefit survival or repro-duction. Most evolutionary theories of low mood view mild depression as adaptive, with major depression being a disordered response at the extreme end of the normal distribution of mood levels (Dowds, 2018; Jang, 2005; Nesse, 2009).

The threat to overall fitness (TOF) model of depression as a stress response postulates that the greatest adversities are those which decrease our chances of passing on our genes to the next generation (Maletic & Raison, 2017). These include death before childbearing age, blocks to accessing sexual partners, death before child-rearing is complete, and death of children before the age of reproduction. In our ancestral envi-ronment (environment of evolutionary adaptedness, EEA), the main threats to children's survival were infections by microbes and other par-asites. TOF theory predicts that infection would be a powerful driver of depression—which is indeed the case. Likewise, our place in the social order had a powerful impact on both survival and reproductive fitness, so it is anticipated that brain areas involved in threat recognition and social interaction are most likely to be implicated in depression. Thus, it is not surprising that it is the three main danger pathways that are implicated in the physiology of depression: the two stress response path-ways (HPA and ANS) and the immune system. Some depressed patients display clinical levels of neurotrophic factors, inflammatory cytokines, monoamine neurotransmitters, or HPA components, or autonomic ner-vous system imbalance. However, there is no single biological marker or combination of them that is found in all cases of depression. Some will lack any of the expected markers while others show various combina-tions and degrees of the markers (ibid.).

The selective value of low mood can be seen in many situations. The depressive pain associated with loss keeps us close to our attachment partners—which is crucial for survival in children and beneficial in adults. Shutdown and withdrawal behaviours in young mammals sep-arated from their mothers aid in their survival by camouflaging them against predators and preserving their energy resources. Depression-like sickness behaviour preserves our limited resources when ill with infections. Sickness and depression behaviours have a lot in common: apathy, irritability, anxiety, exhaustion, altered sleep patterns, poor appe-tite, cognitive difficulties, and even low-grade fever. However, there are differences, and in most cases only depression is associated with despair, guilt, and self-loathing (ibid.).

In more general terms, depressive behaviour mimics threat responses, and may be seen as a continuation of the reaction long after the threat has passed (see Dowds, 2018 for a fuller discussion and references). In summary, selection may have "shaped different subtypes of depression to deal with problems in different domains" (Nesse, 2009, p. 25).

Genetics

Vulnerability to depression depends on complex interactions between genetic make-up, childhood upbringing, and the adult environment. Genetics plays a role in responses to stress, trauma, and the development of depression. Twin and adoption studies show that about 37 per cent of the variation in liability to depression is due to genetic make-up (expressed as a heritability of 37 per cent), the remaining 63 per cent being down to what is called the "environment": that is, all non-genetic factors such as upbringing, diet, education, socio-economic circumstances, etc. (Plomin et al., 2013). Variants of a large number of different genes, each of small effect, combine to generate genetic liability. Heritability varies in different groups, being larger among women, in groups with adolescent onset, and among populations with chronic and severe depression (references in Hammen & Watkins, 2018, p. 94). Interestingly, different symptoms of depression have different heritability patterns (Kendler et al., 2013), indicating again how heterogeneous this syndrome is.

Because individual gene variants have only a small effect on depression, it has proved difficult to identify them and many of the findings have not been replicated in subsequent studies. One approach has examined the impact of candidate genes on depression, particularly when they are tested in a variety of environments (gene-environment interaction). Candidate genes code for endophenotypes (i.e. measures of gene function that increase the risk of psychopathology), rather than any specific diagnosis. In the case of mood disorders, these genes can be expected to play roles in emotional regulation, response to threat and stress, and immune activity. However, a recent meta-analysis examined the role in depression of eighteen candidate genes that have been studied ten times or more. This study was based on sample sizes orders of magnitude larger than earlier research and found that previous conclusions linking these candidate genes to depression were founded on false positive results (Border et al., 2019). *No evidence was found linking any of the candidate gene polymorphisms with depression.* (A polymorphism is a common variation in DNA sequence in a population, similar to an allele.)

A more promising methodology for identifying large numbers of genes of low impact is genome-wide association studies (GWAS) which examine polymorphisms in the entire genome in very large sample sizes. A recent meta-analysis of the three largest of these studies has identified 269 genes and fifteen gene sets associated with depression (Howard et al., 2019). Depression-associated genes included those involved in biological pathways of response to stimuli and neurotransmission, though interestingly not genes linked with the serotonergic system.

It must be borne in mind that individual gene variants generally have only a small impact, and it is the additive combination of alleles, the interaction between different genes, and the interaction between genes and the environment that together explain an individual's susceptibility to depression and/or anxiety. Thus, the influence of genes is moderated by social variables, gender, and environmental adversity. The impact of childhood adversity is more profound and lasting than stress in later life, occurring as it does during the years when the brain and nervous system are being formed. Hundreds of research projects have searched for and purported to find a link between depression and interactions between specific candidate gene variants and adverse experiences in childhood. However, the meta-analysis mentioned above (Border et al., 2019) has shown that the early research was severely underpowered, and in some cases incorrectly analysed. Thus, to date, this research is a history of false positives.

There is substantial overlap between the genes that contribute to different psychopathologies, including 100 per cent overlap (correlation coefficient, $r = 1$) between the genes predisposing to major depression disorder and generalised anxiety disorder (Plomin et al., 2013). Whether an individual develops GAD or MDD is thus down to environmental differences.

Other traits displaying a relatively high genetic correlation with depression include bipolar disorder ($r = 0.33$) and schizophrenia (r = 0.32). The connections here have been shown to be non-causative. Rather the shared genes have pleiotropic effects, that is, they affect several apparently distinct traits (Howard et al., 2019).

Intergenerational transmission of depression

The rates of major depression among relatives of depressed people is about three times higher than a control group, and children of a depressed parent have a 50 per cent chance of developing some kind of psychopathology, including a 20 to 40 per cent chance of becoming depressed (references in Hammen & Watkins, 2018, pp. 94, 182). These children also suffer a variety of problems with health, and cognitive and social development. Both mothers' and fathers' depression have a negative effect on children, though the latter to a lesser degree.

Intergenerational transmission of depression might in principle be explained by genetic or environmental (child rearing) contributions or both. Separating out these two factors is hampered by the problem of gene-environment correlation: here the genes shared between parent and child determine a significant part of the rearing environment. For example, a child's genetically influenced personality trait, like neuroticism or introversion, may evoke a patterned negative response from a parent with the same traits. A children of twins study showed that environmental as well as genetic factors mediated the link between parent and juvenile depression (Silberg et al., 2010). One study (Harold et al., 2011) has disentangled genetic vs environmental factors by sampling families with children conceived through IVF. This generates parent–child dyads where the child is genetically related to the mother only; father only; neither parent; or both parents but with a surrogate intrauterine environment. This research showed that depressed mothers—but not fathers—transmitted depression to genetically unrelated children. Likewise, earlier adoption studies showed associations between child and adolescent outcomes and having a depressed adoptive mother, but no link to depression in the adoptive father (Leve et al., 2010; Tully et al., 2008).

The evidence supports the conclusion that mothers, through their role as primary caregivers, can promote stress and depression or resilience in their children depending on their parenting capacities. Studies of adolescents showed that the link was entirely mediated by family and interpersonal stress (Garber & Cole, 2010; Hammen et al., 2004), and that associations between stress and depression are bidirectional (Hammen et al., 2012), while individual adverse events have a slightly larger impact than shared family environment (references in Hammen & Watkins, 2018, p. 95). The impact of maternal depression promoted first onset in early adolescence, but did not predict adult-onset depression.

Maternal depression has negative impacts on children whether it occurs during pregnancy or postpartum. Mother/infant observation studies revealed depressed mothers being intrusive (critical and irritated) and/or withdrawn and disengaged (references in Hammen & Watkins, 2018, p. 184). Parental depression is usually embedded in a range of psycho-socio-economic stresses such as marital problems, socio-economic disadvantage, poor communication skills, and a generally impaired environment for learning social and problem-solving skills.

Epigenetics

Changes in the environment regulate gene expression through epigenetic modification (e.g. by methylation) of relevant genes, the mechanism underlying gene-environment (G x E) interactions. The early postnatal period of development has a heightened sensitivity to environmental influences, particularly the quality of caregiving (see Chapter 4), and evidence is increasingly emerging that epigenetic marking of the genome may underlie at least some aspects of this process (Roth & Sweatt, 2011). However, it is important to note that because of genetic polymorphisms (variations in DNA sequence between individuals), in many cases experiences that produce a certain outcome in some people do not do so in others.

The work of Michael Meaney and colleagues links neglectful maternal behaviour in rats to stress in their offspring (references in Boyce, 2019; Dowds, 2018; Sweatt et al., 2013). Female pups who were neglected by their own mothers in turn exhibited low nurturance behaviour to their own offspring. The neglectful mothers were not simply genetically programmed to behave this way since they varied in their treatment of individual pups. Furthermore, the transmission of poor parenting across generations was not due to genes held in common, because in cross-fostering experiments the females displayed the pup-licking traits of their foster mothers, rather than their genetic mums.

It turns out that good mothering reduces stress in offspring via epigenetic modification of genes involved in the stress response. Maternal attention decreased methylation of the gene coding for the glucocorticoid receptor (GR) within cells of the pups' hippocampus, thereby increasing GR expression and downregulating the stress response (see later in this chapter). The reverse pattern was observed in humans maltreated in childhood, who later took their own lives (McGowan et al., 2009). In these cases, increased methylation of the GR gene was accounted for by early life adversity rather than whether the individuals were suffering from depression when they committed suicide.

Childhood abuse is associated with the occurrence of major depression and other psychopathologies in adulthood, and a number of areas of the brain (including the prefrontal cortex, corpus callosum, amygdala, and hippocampus) as well as the HPA stress response system are impacted by these experiences (references in Roth & Sweatt, 2011). Maltreatment of rats during the first week of life resulted in methylation of the gene coding for brain-derived neurotrophic factor (BDNF, which mediates neural function and plasticity) in the prefrontal cortex (ibid.). The hypermethylated DNA persisted into adulthood and was associated with reduced expression of this gene. The maltreated females displayed the same pattern of abuse towards offspring as they themselves had experienced, and the pups had the same BDNF methylation pattern as their mothers. What was the basis of this intergenerational transmission of abusive behaviour? Was it behavioural or epigenetic? It turned out that fostering the pups to non-stressed females did not completely reverse the methylation pattern, showing that maternal behaviour was not the only explanation. There are two possibilities for the apparent inheritance of the methylation pattern. Either the BDNF gene was methylated in the mothers' germline cells and then acquired by the pups, or the foetal gene was methylated *in utero* perhaps because of the mother's anxiety while pregnant. Epigenetic programming has also been demonstrated that affects HPA activity in mice after mother-infant separation and following prenatal stress (references in Roth & Sweatt, 2011).

Children born to Holocaust survivors but conceived after this trauma displayed a heightened stress response system that was linked to epigenetic modification of stress response genes (Bowers & Yehuda, 2016; Yehuda et al., 2016). They are excessively prone to mental health problems including depression, anxiety, and PTSD as well as chronic physical illness (Boyce, 2019).

Many of these studies (e.g. Yehuda et al., 2016) have appeared to demonstrate the intergenerational transmission of these epigenetic markers. However, in humans and other mammals, all or virtually all of these modifications are erased in the germ line, and serious doubt has been cast on the validity of some of these research studies. Their statistical methodology has been shown to be inadequate for the conclusions drawn, and such transgenerational transmission lacks any plausible mechanism. Paper after paper has purported to show strange, inconsistent patterns of inheritance of epigenetic modifications, and yet—unlike other dramatic and unexpected results in science—there has been no progression in the work, just more tenuous illustrations (Mitchell, 2018a, 2018b).

There is no doubt, however, that the impact of the environment on mental and physical diseases, physiological processes, overreactive stress responses, and trauma are passed on from generation to generation. For example, exercise in one generation has cardiovascular and metabolic benefits for descendants, while the impact of the Dutch famine of 1944–45 was felt by at least two subsequent generations in rates of obesity, diabetes, neurodegenerative disorders, etc. (Boyce, 2019). If we rule out the transmission of epigenetic modifications of the DNA through the germline, what other possible ways might an individual's experience of trauma or famine be passed on to their children and grandchildren who have not themselves had these experiences? There are many possibilities, including material inheritance (of poverty or wealth). During our most formative years, we inhabit the same environment as our parents, and through modelling we learn the same patterns of behaviour, relating, affect regulation, and other forms of emotional processing (experiential transmission). Another likely possibility is that foetal DNA is methylated *in utero* in response to the mother's ongoing stress, trauma, depression, and other experiences she has undergone in her life prior to becoming pregnant.

Epigenetic programming within the foetus has been documented in humans (references in Roth & Sweatt, 2011). The glucocorticoid receptor gene involved in regulating the HPA stress response was methylated in the foetuses of mothers with high levels of depression and anxiety during the third trimester, while babies delivered by C-section had high levels of global DNA methylation. With humans it is not ethically possible to remove cells of the central nervous system for DNA methylation analysis. Therefore, the methylation patterns in these cases were detected in cord blood cells and leucocytes respectively, and it is not known if these peripheral cells reflect methylation patterns within the CNS.

Epigenetic modification induced by early life experience can be experimentally reversed via pharmacological (e.g. methylation-inhibiting drugs) or behavioural routes, but the research is a long way from clinical application as yet.

The role of temperament: orchids and dandelions

There are individual variations in the response to adverse circumstances and the risk for developing depression as a consequence. Among the five OCEAN personality traits, high levels of neuroticism (the N in OCEAN) correlate with an increased likelihood of depression (Plomin et al., 2013). Among the traits which are co-morbid with and genetically correlate with depression, neuroticism was the only one with a putative bidirectional causal effect (Howard et al., 2019). Neuroticism, like the other OCEAN personality traits, is roughly half genetic and half determined by the environment.

Research into so-called "dandelion" and "orchid" children also shows that not all temperaments are equally vulnerable to stress and depression. The intensity of stress responses in children follows a normal curve, with some being unusually sensitive, others unusually resilient, and the majority in the mid-range. Newborn babies are routinely tested for activity, respiration, pulse rate, and reflexes, all of which are controlled by the ANS, and the scores reveal the body's adaptation to the stress of the birth process. This stress resilience at birth was found to predict teacher-reported developmental vulnerability at age five. The 20 per cent of children at the extreme end of stress sensitivity experience the majority of physical and psychological illnesses and this childhood vulnerability extends into adulthood. These children were found to be hypersensitive in a range of stress tests assessing resilience to psychosocial, physical, emotional, and cognitive stressors (Boyce, 2019). Reactions were tested via measures reflecting the HPA (salivary cortisol

levels) reaction, the fight-flight (HRV for PNS and timing of the car-
diac cycle for the SNS) stress response, and both acting together (e.g.
blood pressure and heart rate).The more resilient children—nicknamed
dandelions by Boyce—thrive in almost any environment, whereas the
highly reactive ones (orchids) do badly in adverse circumstances, but
exceptionally well (vital, creative, and successful) in supportive nurturing environments. Harsh circumstances in life ranged from harsh
parenting, impoverished neighbourhoods, violence experienced or wit-
nessed, and maltreatment, neglect, and abuse. The highly stress-reactive
children were exceptionally permeable and sensitive to the nature of
their social worlds, and were either the sickest *or the healthiest*, depending on their home and social environments. One test starkly revealed
the difference in sensitivity to the psychosocial conditions. When inter-
viewed by two researchers, one kind and interested, the other rude and
grim, the dandelion children were able to remember and describe an
incident from two weeks previously equally well with the two interview-
ers, whereas the orchids remembered even more details with the "nice"
researcher but couldn't remember anything at all when faced with the
nasty interlocutor. The orchids were also found to have a far greater
capacity to resist temptation, as well as greater activity in the right prefrontal cortex, the side involved in emotional regulation, impulse control, and planning.

It is likely that an individual's resilience to stress is caused by their
particular genetic make-up interacting with their environment—
experience in the womb, attachment security, and so on. Unfortunately,
the studies which have attempted to identify some of these genes were
all underpowered, so a lot more work is needed before definitive conclusions can be reached.

Orchid children who grow up in non-supportive environments are
prone to externalising (e.g. aggression or defiance) and internalising
(e.g. depression and anxiety) behaviours (Boyce, 2019). Orchids have
more active right hemispheres than dandelions, and frontal lobe activation in the right hemisphere is associated with depression and anxiety (Cozolino, 2010). All of this suggests that for orchids and depressed
people it takes more effort to keep their thoughts and feelings stable
and regulated. Symptoms of depression and anxiety in children were

found to be correlated with a highly reactive fight or flight system, and were linked with a low social rank in the classroom hierarchy in cases where the teachers ignored, or even fostered, dominance of the weak by the strong. On the other hand, when teachers undermined the formation of hierarchies with egalitarian teaching approaches, low social rank did not give rise to depressive symptoms.

Stress and the environment

Stress, whether physical (e.g. illness) or psychosocial (e.g. loss of attachment partner; humiliation/ loss of status), is a primary risk factor for depression. Some of these stresses can be partly self-generated, and there is a genetic link between the tendency to make stressful life choices and vulnerability to depression. Genes contribute to neuroticism, which generates stress. Early environmental experience can also lead us to be unconsciously drawn to stressful situations: children who were abused, neglected, or traumatised (e.g. by death of a parent) develop personalities that increase the risk of interpersonal conflict and of making life choices that generate stress (references in Maletic & Raison, 2017, Chapter 3).

Does adult environmental stress actually cause depression, or does childhood adversity leave the adult more prone to making stressful life "choices" and also, independently, to be more liable to depression? This question has been addressed by comparing societies with high vs low levels of stress and depression and where the main stressors are not individual and self-generated. The research revealed that there is a causal and dose-response relationship between environmental adversity and MDD (ibid.).

The most powerful depressogenic losses are abstract and people are often willing to be hurt or face death rather than lose face by being defeated or humiliated. These losses are worst when they are inescapable, or perceived as such: "Environmental adversities, especially those of a dependent, humiliating, defeating, socially rejecting, and entrapping nature, are causally related to depression" (Maletic & Raison, 2017, p. 68). Furthermore, it is perception of adversity—for example, *how* you interpret being fired from your job and *how* you perceive it shaping your future—rather than the nature of the event that is depressogenic.

Thus, depression is a mind/body state of perceiving oneself in a position of loss or defeat; and it is a state that increases the chances that the individual will behave in ways that make loss and defeat more likely.

Stress is not, however, a sufficient cause for depression. It is possible that it is not even necessary, though that is harder to judge since what may seem like a minor stress to one person may be major to another. However, stress is certainly a major contributor to depression—as well as to a wide range of other psychological and physical ailments. Maletic and Raison conclude that "Stress may cause one lifelong health condition that manifests in different ways at different ages and in different people depending on their other vulnerabilities" (2017, p. 110).

Stress responses

There are two stress response systems, both of which are initiated by the amygdala triggering the hypothalamus. The HPA cascade results in the release of the stress hormone, cortisol; while the fight, flight, freeze system of the autonomic nervous system (ANS) releases epinephrine and norepinephrine from the adrenal glands. The stress and threat hormones then go on to alter the body's physiology as appropriate for arousal or shutdown by monitoring and regulating numerous physiological processes, including blood glucose levels, blood pressure, heart rate, the immune system, and digestion.

The ANS is a rapid response system, and epinephrine release occurs much faster than the production of cortisol by the HPA, but the two systems cross-communicate, with the HPA also activating the norepinephrine circuitry and the ANS regulating HPA reactivity (Maletic & Raison, 2017).

The ANS

The ANS is the part of the nervous system that controls the internal organs such as the adrenal glands, heart, lungs, diaphragm, and gastrointestinal system. It has two divisions: the sympathetic nervous system (SNS) which increases energy expenditure and prepares the body for action; while the parasympathetic nervous system (PNS) enhances body activities that gain and conserve energy—activities that have been labelled: rest and digest; feed and breed; tend and befriend. In response to danger, the ANS reacts sequentially. First, PNS tone is withdrawn. If this is inadequate to the perceived threat, the SNS is activated with the release of the neurotransmitter norepinephrine. Then, perhaps thirty seconds later, epinephrine is released from the adrenal glands, the heart rate increases and the body physiology is switched towards arousal. In depression the ANS is imbalanced in the direction of arousal mediated by the SNS, and withdrawal regulated by the PNS (ibid.), and we explore this in more detail in the next chapter.

Hypothalamic–pituitary–adrenal (HPA) axis

The HPA cascade can be activated by either environmental stress or elevated levels of pro-inflammatory cytokines (Carabotti et al., 2015). The axis is initiated by the amygdala signalling the hypothalamus to secrete corticotrophin-releasing hormone (CRH). CRH acts upwards into the brain where it functions as a neurotransmitter to promote states of fear, vigilance, and enhanced memory of the stress trigger. Downwards into the body, CRH serves as a hormone to act on the pituitary gland to release ACTH, which then triggers the adrenal glands to produce the glucocorticoid hormone, cortisol. CRH also reinforces other activators of the SNS via its effects on the brainstem. All cells contain receptors for binding cortisol, which then goes on to up- or down-regulate expression of a battery of genes. The combined consequences are that the body is primed for the fight-flight response via a range of physiological changes including increased blood pressure and glucose production, anti-inflammatory action, and redirection of immune cells (Maletic & Raison, 2017).

Depression correlates with increased cortisol levels, less of a diurnal fluctuation in the hormone, and reduced sensitivity to negative feedback that mediates the return to basal, non-threat levels of cortisol. Cortisol operates a negative feedback loop and switches off the HPA axis at three control points: the hypothalamus, the pituitary, and the adrenal glands. For this reason, cortisol is not only a sign of stress, but a mediator of the anti-stress response. This is what makes it difficult to interpret the finding that cortisol levels are elevated in depression. These high levels are often linked with problems in switching off the HPA axis because chronic exposure to cortisol causes receptors to become less efficient. After a lengthy discussion of many strands of evidence, Maletic and Raison conclude that "It is this inability of chronically high glucocorticoids to optimise inhibitory feedback that explains why prolonged exposure to high levels of glucocorticoids promotes depression, not because cortisol is a depressogenic substance in and of itself" (2017, p. 216).

The HPA response is programmed in the womb and during an early critical postnatal period as shown by a number of prospective studies (Gerhardt, 2015). Children living with stressed mothers at the age of four had high levels of cortisol if their mothers were stressed or depressed when they were infants, but not if they spent their early months under low stress conditions. Children who *did* experience stress in babyhood didn't have high *basal* levels of cortisol, but they were programmed to react more strongly to later difficulties (Essex et al., 2002). Likewise, cortisol reactivity in adolescence was found to correlate with an absence of warmth and responsiveness in early childhood (Hackman et al., 2013). Research on Romanian orphans showed that only those adopted before the age of four months were able to reset their HPA system to an unstressed level of reactivity. After the age of six months the cortisol response stabilises and remains consistent (Lewis & Ramsay, 1995).

PTSD is associated with low levels of cortisol, possibly due to a more powerful negative feedback loop. Women who were pregnant at the time of the 9/11 attack on the World Trade Center reacted in two ways: those who went on to suffer PTSD were found to have low levels of cortisol, whereas those who did not had normal, moderate levels of the stress hormone (Yehuda et al., 2005). The babies of the PTSD mothers also had low levels of cortisol, suggesting that the HPA system is partially programmed in the womb.

There are implications for the process of therapy in this early setting of the HPA stress response in the womb and the first six months after birth. We must be realistic about the degree to which therapy can improve resilience in clients with early trauma, and help them set realistic targets for themselves: they can learn to limit their exposure to stress, but may have to curb their ego's desire for great achievement in highly stressful endeavours. This is particularly difficult for young people to accept and they may have to grieve the loss of their dreams for the future.

Inflammation

In the environment in which human beings originally evolved, the major threat for children was infection. Thus, infection must be classed as a significant stress which leaves the individual open to depression (Maletic & Raison, 2017). The most vulnerable entry sites for infection are the gastrointestinal system, the respiratory system, and the skin, and these boundary zones are protected by a range of immune cells—macrophages, neutrophils, and dendritic cells. Receptors on these cells bind to molecules found on the surface of pathogens and activate immune processes that are as widespread and non-selectively damaging as possible: this is the inflammatory response. Apart from this innate, non-specific immune system, mammals also have a more specific system of acquired immunity comprising the T and B cell responses.

Chemicals called cytokines, which signal the brain and body to fight infection, are produced by the sentry cells of the innate immune system as well as by T lymphocytes and B lymphocytes. Cytokine activation in the body induces the brain to start producing them, and their presence in the brain causes organs of the body to make more cytokines.

Inflammation and depression

Immune responses are constrained by regulatory cells which, if they underperform, can promote inflammatory and autoimmune conditions, or if they overperform (immune suppression) can increase vulnerability to cancer. Of most importance to us in the context of depression is the evidence suggesting that "Suboptimal immunoregulatory functioning may be a common feature of Major Depression and may in fact contribute to the proinflammatory state often observed in MDD" (Maletic & Raison, 2017, p. 187).

Cytokine levels well below concentrations needed to induce sickness are sufficient to generate depression, and cytokine antagonists abolish these behaviours. It is the cytokine activity rather than infection itself that promotes low mood, and there is increasing evidence that cytokines induce depression by activating inflammation.

It turns out that psychosocial stress produces changes in the immune system that resemble those seen during infection, and the evidence is building that inflammation is the mediating factor in responses to adversity. Maletic and Raison (2017) list risk factors for depression that also increase inflammation, and they suggest that the proliferation of some of these may explain the dramatic increase in MDD over the last fifty years. The inflammatory stresses that have increased include: psychosocial stress, sedentary lifestyle, obesity, social isolation, consumption of processed foods, smoking, and air pollution. Among the risk factors, only medical illness has reduced, while some like seasonal change have remained the same. Both acute and chronic stress and early life adversity produce inflammation and depression, and almost every risk factor for depression (including lack of exercise and sleep, processed foods and obesity) increases peripheral inflammatory signals. However, it is clear that inflammation is neither necessary nor sufficient to cause MDD. Nevertheless, there is a subtype of depression characterised by high levels of inflammatory cytokines. The two related factors of obesity and early life adversity are particularly correlated with this subtype: both are linked with high levels of inflammation as well as increased risk of depression as a response to inflammation (Maletic & Raison, 2017).

Gut microbiota

Bidirectional communication between the intestine and emotional and cognitive centres in the brain forms the gut-brain axis. This is mediated by the central, enteric, and autonomic nervous systems as well as the endocrine and immune systems and the HPA stress response (Carabotti et al., 2015). Within the gut is a huge population of bacteria and other microbes—about 1,000 different species—referred to collectively as the gut microbiota or microbiome, and they play a role in influencing the gut-brain interactions (see Dowds, 2018 for a fuller discussion). The profile of these bacteria is altered by stress and diet, and decreased diversity and imbalance of species in the microbiome can in turn generate stress, depression, and anxiety (Foster & Neufeld, 2013). Indeed, when faecal microbiota from depressed human patients were transplanted into rats, they generated depression and anxiety behaviours (Kelly et al., 2016).

A healthy diet and consumption of probiotics (including *Lactobacillus* and *Bifidobacterium* species) helps both prevent and treat depression. Foods high in fat (which contributes to leaky gut and inflammation) and sugar, and low in fibre, reduce microbial diversity and are associated with depression, while diets high in plants, complex carbohydrates, and fermented food support microbial diversity, including anti-inflammatory bacteria, and promote good mental health (Dash et al., 2015).

Summary

Predisposition to depression is partially determined by genetic make-up (37 per cent), while childhood adversity accounts for most of the vulnerability. There is substantial overlap in the genetic variation that confers liability to many kinds of psychopathology, and depression and anxiety are the same phenomenon genetically. Some personality types (those high in neuroticism) and some temperaments (so-called "orchids") are more vulnerable to stress, depression, and anxiety.

Depression is associated with a number of changes in both HPA and ANS responses to threat, including increased cortisol levels and the ANS tending towards SNS arousal and PNS withdrawal. The HPA stress response is programmed in the womb and the first few months of life, thus generating a lack of stress resilience in people who encountered adversity at that time.

Depression can be triggered by physical illness including infection, as well as by psychosocial stresses, and the common mediator in one subtype of the disorder appears to be inflammation. The role of gut microbes and diet in depression may be at least partially governed by inflammatory effects.

CHAPTER 3

An application of neuroscience

No area of science has made a more crucial contribution to therapy theory and practice than neuroscience, particularly our knowledge of the ANS and polyvagal system. This is because it shows how early threats—including threats to the attachment system—are not just engraved in, but actually shaped the development of the individual's nervous system. Depression is linked with multiple or ongoing adverse experiences in childhood, which usually originate in relational threat of the abusive, rejecting, or severely neglectful kind—including insecure attachment (most traumatically of the disorganised variety) with caregivers, or being at the mercy of abusive adults or children (bullying), or losing a parent. The result of these threats is to lay down patterns in relation to other people such as hypervigilance, avoidance, submission, and lack of boundaries. An understanding of how the nervous system has been primed by early experiences to react to danger helps us to understand how to work with trauma, depression, and anxiety.

The ANS and the polyvagal system

The ANS responds to conditions of threat or safety by regulating the inner organs and glands, including the adrenal glands (see Chapter 2).

The cranial nerves in the brainstem link arousal in the body to the brain, and control the focus of the eyes (broad vs narrow focus), facial expression, hearing, and the vestibular system.

In a situation of danger, the body's physiology switches into the high arousal (mediated by the SNS) needed for the fight or flight response. If the individual is too powerless to fight or flee (e.g. the child with an abusive parent), they submit to the aggressor and may enter a state of shock, or ultimately into a freeze state of immobilisation (see Table 3.1). This calls for inhibition of arousal, which is mediated by the parasympathetic branch of the ANS.

Table 3.1

Threat	Power in relation to threat	Response	Somatic state	ANS activation
+	++	Fight	Hyperarousal	SNS
+	+	Flight	Hyperarousal	SNS
+	–	Freeze	Immobilisation	PNS: dorsal vagus
–	n/a	Social engagement	Calm alertness	PNS: ventral vagus

The tenth cranial nerve is the vagus nerve—actually a bundle of nerves—which regulates the parasympathetic nervous system (PNS). It travels downwards to the organs of the body and upwards to the throat, eyes, and ears through its connection with other cranial nerves. It has two pathways: the more primitive, unmyelinated dorsal vagus that regulates the above collapse or immobilisation responses; and—a branch that evolved with mammals—the myelinated ventral vagus that mediates a state of alert calmness when we feel both safe and connected (Dana, 2018). The three states mediated through the SNS, dorsal vagus, and ventral vagus manifest different physiologies, experiences, and behaviours. The ventral vagus controls the heart, lungs, and airways, while the dorsal regulates the organs of digestion including the liver, pancreas, and spleen, as well as the heart and lungs (Rosenberg, 2017). It is only when the ventral vagus is activated that the social engagement system is switched on: here the individual is in their optimum arousal zone, or window of tolerance (Ogden et al., 2006). The brain integrates signals from the ventral vagus with somatosensory nerves that control muscles of the eyes, face, and also the inner ear to tune it for the sound frequency of the human voice.

For contemporary humankind, the nature of the threat to our well-being is rarely the proximity of a predator species, though we may have this experience when we encounter a viper or rattlesnake when out for a country walk. Most of our current experience of danger comes from other members of our own species, and what is threatened is usually our sense of self and/or our place in the social order rather than our lives or even livelihoods. Being bullied at school or work or attacked on social media, being lonely or friendless, surviving in non-hostile but unattuned relationships, being gaslighted by a malignant narcissist, worrying that we are being tricked or manipulated—all are threats that trigger the SNS or dorsal vagus. Our responses to social dangers are usually not physical, but may include verbal aggression (fight); social avoidance or withdrawal (flight); compliance (the beginning of giving up); or a plunge into extreme depression (emotional freeze).

Our sensitivity to social dangers depends on our past experiences, particularly those in childhood. In relatively benign situations where we expect reciprocal I-thou connections but those expectations are violated (e.g. we get a blank stare, or in Tronick's term, a "still face", instead of interactive engagement), we experience what Porges calls "biological rudeness", and we feel unsafe (Dana, 2018). A relationship that involves co-regulation (see Chapter 4) generates a state of safety for the participants, whereas the absence of this—for example, in disconnected people or those living with hostile or non-attuned others—creates loneliness, unsafeness, and health problems including depression.

People who had attuned parents capable of consistently reading and meeting their needs have experienced co-regulation and thus develop a mental model of relationships that is secure: in the words of Daniel Siegel, they feel seen, soothed, and safe. For those who experienced caregiving that was rejecting or emotionally distant (avoidant); inconsistent or intrusive (ambivalent); or frightening, confusing, or fearful (disorganised), their attachment model is insecure and they do not feel seen or soothed, while those in the disorganised group feel sufficiently unsafe for them to be classed as suffering from developmental or relational trauma. Thus, the securely attached are less likely than the insecure to be driven out of the ventral vagal state of thriving into SNS or dorsal vagal survival modes. For the insecurely attached, on the other hand, relational dynamics that re-stimulate the old neglect or abuse embedded in their nervous systems can easily tip the individual into fight, flight, or freeze responses, or even in extreme cases into breakdown. These triggers might include the experience of not being seen, heard, or understood, of being controlled, manipulated, criticised, judged, excluded, or of meeting a wall of denial about the incongruent emotional dynamics in a group or workplace. Of course, such triggering is taking place below the level of the conscious mind. Therefore suggestions to be less sensitive or to take a more detached view are futile and likely to be experienced as invalidating, thus creating a further trigger.

The three steps of the ladder

There is a hierarchy of response in the ANS, according to the evolutionary age of the three neural pathways: the dorsal vagus being the oldest, then the SNS, followed by the most recent ventral vagus. At the summit of this evolutionary ladder (ventral vagus), our heart rate is regulated, our breath is deep and slow, and we are capable of "seeing" other people (i.e. mentalizing), connecting to ourselves and the world, and tuning out distracting noises. In this state we are active and interested, we can concentrate, self-regulate, and balance work and play. Those whose lives are dominated by ventral vagal experiences are likely to have good health (heart, immune system, digestion, and sleep) and well-being (Dana, 2018).

You feel insulted or judged by one of your peers and become angry. You feel anxious because of the threat of emotional abandonment (common for the ambivalently attached) or a demand for intimacy (prevalent among the avoidantly attached). The angry (fight) and anxious (flight) responses to threat are mediated by the neural circuits of the SNS. The heart rate speeds up, the breath becomes rapid and shallow, our eyes and ears scan the environment for danger, the eyes becoming focused, the ears now tuned to low frequency sounds of danger or high frequency sounds of distress. In this state, the ability to read the human face is compromised, and a neutral face can be perceived as angry or dangerous (ibid.). If we habitually inhabit such a state, the health consequences can include heart disease, high blood pressure, high levels of cholesterol, sleep problems, weight gain, poor memory, muscle tension, and an impaired immune system.

When the environment is unsafe but we cannot respond via the SNS (e.g. we can't get away from or rage against an abusive boss because we have no confidence we could find another job) we may fall into the dorsal vagal pathway and conserve our energy from fruitless and/or dangerous expenditure. Underlying our apparent compliant behaviour is a state of despair, collapse, and dissociation, where we are unable to think clearly or act in a focused way, where we feel numb and abandoned, and where the world seems "empty, dead and dark" (Dana, 2018, p. 12). In a state of extreme terror or pain, we may defecate, faint, or dissociate (Porges, 2018). Health consequences following on from prolonged dorsal vagal living can include chronic fatigue, fibromyalgia, digestive problems, low blood pressure, type 2 diabetes, weight gain, memory impairment, isolation, and depression.

In responding to challenges in the environment we follow a downward hierarchy, starting with the most recent of the autonomic pathways (the ventral vagus), followed by the SNS, followed by the most primitive dorsal vagus (Porges, 2018). On encountering a potential rapist, a woman might try to reason him out of it (ventral vagal pathway); if that fails she might make a run for it, or knee him in the groin (SNS); and if these tactics fail she may dissociate (dorsal vagus).

Mixed states

Some experiences involve interactions between two autonomic states. When the ventral vagus is coupled with the SNS or dorsal vagus, the individual does not sink into a defensive state, and the range of behaviours and feelings is expanded. When the vagal brake is flexible, it can relax—allowing mobilisation into the SNS—and then re-engage before a threat response comes into action. This combination of activity in the SNS and ventral vagus permits social play, competitive sport, and sexual foreplay. A well-loved and trusted father can throw his child in the air and elicit delight rather than fear because the ventral vagus is activated in father—and therefore in the child. Play is one of the basic emotions that is suppressed in depression, and learning to play is one way out of this fixed state. Play is not only a source of positive emotions, but also of spontaneity, flexibility, and creativity, as Winnicott noted.

When the ventral vagus works together with the dorsal we can experience immobilisation without fear and shutdown, resulting in a *being* state of stillness and tranquillity. Intimacy and love are made possible in this blended state when close contact is interpreted as safe and welcome. However, in the case of people who associate closeness with threat, the social engagement system is not switched on when a person who is otherwise experienced as safe seeks intimacy. Therapy with such clients requires attuned contact to help them develop awareness and tolerance of that edge between safety and danger, as we will see in Chapter 7.

Neuroception and interoception

Porges defines neuroception as "a neural process, distinct from perception, capable of distinguishing environmental and visceral features that are safe, dangerous, or life-threatening" (2018, p. 58). These reflexive shifts in the ANS incorporate interoception, which is our sensing of our internal physiology (Dana, 2018). Colloquial expressions reflect the connections between emotions and body sensations when we say: I feel gutted; he had a gut feeling; she spoke of a broken heart, a knot in the stomach, or a lump in the throat. Body sensations, particularly in the throat, chest, stomach, and gut, form the basis of what Gendlin (1996) has called the felt sense of our lived experience. If we attend to these somatic signals, they provide us with information about survival or joy that should—in a state of health—influence our behaviour and decision making. The information flows in both directions, with our physiology influencing our thoughts and our thoughts changing our physiology (Porges, 2018)—encouraging news for therapists.

We experience a state of anxiety when the stomach is knotted, breathing is shallow and rapid, eye focus is narrow and intense, and hearing is acute—as is the case when the SNS is activated. If we spend a prolonged time in a dorsal vagal state, we experience this as a state of depression where we have no energy, and feel numb, exhausted, and unable to relate to others. Of course, we all shuttle back and forth between the three states, depending on the level of safety or danger in the environment, and it is only when we spend prolonged periods of time in a single state that we can be said to have a fixed mood such as depression. For the majority of people with depression who also suffer from chronic anxiety, the SNS and dorsal vagus are being triggered in alternation.

Many clients cannot activate their defence systems in threatening situations. They are unaware of and find it hard to tune into their felt sense, and respond to people and situations with ingrained patterns of behaviour that habitually place them in risky or stressful reruns of old experiences. For example, one self-employed man repeatedly agreed a zero-profit fee for work, while ignoring his body's alarm bells in the form of a sinking feeling in his heart and a knot in his stomach. Conversely, many traumatised clients cannot inhibit their hypervigilant defence systems, even in safe environments.

The social engagement system and the window of tolerance

The social engagement system enables human beings to communicate flexibly and with potentially great subtlety because the ventral vagus controls looking, emotional expression, hearing (by filtering out background noise), prosody, head tilting and turning, as well as regulating the heart rate without activating the SNS (Porges, 2003). We can move easily between enthusiastic conversation and calm, thoughtful listening as we take turns in social communication. The system thus promotes flexible adaptation, while maintaining our arousal within the window of tolerance.

The window of tolerance is the degree of arousal, neither too little or too much, in which we are capable of processing and integrating experience—perceptions, emotions, body sensations, thoughts, and memories. People with a broad window of tolerance can "cope with greater extremes of arousal and can process complex and stimulating information [internal or external] more effectively. People with a narrow window experience fluctuations as unmanageable and dysregulating" (Ogden et al., 2006, p. 28). A related concept is the response threshold: when this is low, little stimulus is required to arouse the nervous system; when it is high, more input is needed. The optimum threshold is one high enough to tolerate environmental complexity and stimulation, and low enough to perceive subtle changes. Thresholds vary between individuals depending on numerous factors including temperament, previous experience, and the nature of the stimulus (e.g. intellectual vs emotional).

Many depressed people have suffered relational or other kinds of trauma. Traumatised individuals often have a narrow and rigid window of tolerance, being easily overwhelmed (hyperaroused) by input (e.g. noise, memories, social interactions), or on the other hand becoming numbed out or dissociated (hypoaroused) in response to what to others might seem a moderate level of stimulus. They often have exceptionally low or high thresholds of response, or they fluctuate between the two. For example, they may sometimes be unaware of traffic bearing down on them, while at other times they might be highly anxious about trivial aspects of physical safety. In therapy, an individual can learn to recognise the triggers for hypo- or hyperarousal, recognise the somatic signs, and find out which physical actions (breathing, supporting the back, grounding with the feet or with eye contact) return him to his window of tolerance. It is axiomatic that clients must process traumatic experience within their window of tolerance; otherwise they will either fail to integrate the past, or—at the other extreme—they may be re-traumatised by the therapy itself.

Emotional homeostasis

The goal of emotional homeostasis and indeed of therapy is to return us to the social engagement system: when the ventral vagus is on-line, the heart is connected with how we look, listen, and speak, so that our non-verbal communication is congruent with our words and we communicate warmth, understanding, and sensitivity. The ventral vagus— through the vagal brake—suppresses the heartbeat from its intrinsic rate of 90 beats/minute to about 72 beats/minute, and gives us flexibility to respond to the energy needs of the situation (heart rate variability, HRV). It is only when danger exceeds the capacity of the HRV to modulate in a moment-by-moment manner that the metabolically costly SNS is activated (Maletic & Raison, 2017). Activation of the ventral vagus (e.g. via safe social engagement) puts the brakes on the SNS (and HPA axis) and dorsal vagus, and reduces inflammation. People with an avoidant attachment style have decreased HRV (Mikulincer & Shaver, 2019). In general those with developmental trauma—who did not experience adequate co-regulation—have a reduced capacity to exercise the vagal brake and regulate their emotions. In therapy they can practise this through intentionally moving between activated and calm states: self-regulation emerges out of co-regulation.

Deb Dana claims that recovery from shutdown requires moving up the evolutionary timeline from the dorsal vagus into the SNS and only then into the ventral vagus (2018, p. 32). Thus exercise, which stimulates the SNS, can help bring people out of depression, which is a dorsal vagal state. Stanley Rosenberg, on the other hand, maintains that it is not necessary to go through stress (SNS) to get to social engagement. Rather, "Ventral vagal activity moves a person directly from shutdown and emotional depression all the way up to a ventral vagal state" (2017, p. 53).

Our neuroception systems are constantly searching for cues of safety or danger, primarily through what we see and hear. In particular, we scan the eyes and cheeks of the other for the degree of mobility and aliveness: do we see soft receptiveness, a focused stare, or empty absence? With respect to sound, it is not the words used, but rather the tone, frequency, duration, intensity, and rhythm that imply safety or threat. All therapists, whatever their orientation, must remember that it is these somatic signals, rather than words, that carry the real—that is, emotional—communication.

Depression and the polyvagal system

Depression's relationship to the ANS is not yet as clearly defined as its connection to the HPA axis. Nevertheless, many kinds of evidence indicate that MDD is characterised by vagal PNS withdrawal and SNS activation (Maletic & Raison, 2017).

Shock is characterised by intense dorsal vagal activity resulting in extreme shutdown, while less extreme but chronic immobilisation with fear (Rosenberg, 2017) may accompany feelings of depression. Many people who suffer depression also feel acute anxiety, anger, stress, or agitation as they switch back and forth between the dorsal vagus and the activated response to threat of the SNS.

Vogt (2018) has categorised degrees of relational trauma according to degrees of abuse and control exerted over a subordinate or dependent person (e.g. a child or prisoner) by another who has power over them (e.g. a parent or gaoler). At the extreme end of the scale, there is total abuse of power by the person in charge and severe trauma in the subordinate individual. If, on the other hand, the parent respects the child's boundaries and relates to him with warmth and empathy, the child's ventral vagus is stimulated and he can experience joy, well-being, and curiosity. In the middle of the abuse of power scale, the parent dominates the child through psychological or physical violence so that the SNS becomes activated and the child lives in a state of flight, fight, and panic. At the far end of the scale (stage 7) the victim of extreme violence such as torture has submitted to the abuser, and there is total breakdown in psychological boundaries. If the individual survives, he remains in a state of death-feigning paralysis with dissociative amnesia about the trauma.

Children of parents who rule by verbal, physical, sexual, or psychological (e.g. emotional blackmail) violence are located at stage 5 on the scale. In this class Vogt also includes children with a depressed mother or addicted father who—because of their attachment needs—give up their need for healthy boundaries and apparently align themselves with the parent. These individuals are caught between the flight and panic of the SNS and the submission, shock, and freeze of the dorsal vagus.

The "good" child is often tragically stunted and deprived. Paula, who presented with acute anxiety, was reluctant to take antidepressants for the condition. The daughter of a depressed and manipulative widowed mother, Paula has failed to develop emotional separation from her. Any disappointment, grief, or loneliness on her mother's part has to be fixed by Paula with daily phone calls, access to grandchildren, or having mother to stay. If she fails to read mother's mind or appreciate her "sacrifices", Paula is crippled with guilt and self-loathing. Her anxiety concerns the impossibility of pleasing everyone as well as failing to meet the goals prescribed for her generation by social media. She swings back and forth between this anxiety and depression due to the absence of any authentic libido to drive her life forward. Once she became aware of the emotional blackmail, her guilt became saturated with resentment as well. Her mother never recovered from her husband's death when

Paula was two, so that Paula in turn is now incapable of making her own life. She is heartbroken with loneliness and the discovery that being a good, compliant daughter all her life has yielded nothing but complaints from her mother or irritation and impatience from others. Moreover, she has the usual double-binds of people whose boundaries have been infringed: she cannot ask for help because that would further increase her load of guilt because of all that she would owe the other and the power that would give them over her.

Conclusion

Threatening and stressful events—particularly those encountered in relationships during the formative years of childhood—imprint the nervous system with characteristic patterns. They cause the ANS to remain easily provoked into SNS arousal or dorsal vagus immobilisation, as well as the various gradations between them, including shock and panic reactions and submission to others. These are the patterns that dominate people suffering from depression and anxiety. The polyvagal theory shows us ways of working towards gradually widening the client's window of tolerance towards relational (and other) stimuli, as we will see in Chapter 7. It also demonstrates the conditions in which we are available for social engagement, and how safe relationships can help us emerge from states of over- or under-arousal.

CHAPTER 4

Childhood origins and adult triggers

Depression as an evolutionary adaptation to psychosocial adversity

The threat to overall fitness model argues that triggers for depression coincide with threats to survival or reproductive success (Maletic & Raison, 2017). The environment of evolutionary adaptedness (EEA) is the Stone Age environment in which humans evolved and whose selective pressures we still carry in our genes. The main threats in the EEA, according to Maletic and Raison, were: (a) infection; and (b) social isolation, exclusion, or rejection. Chapters 2 and 3 discussed infection and the immune response as well as the neuroscience of threat responses. Here I want to explore which psychosocial adversities trigger depression, and how low mood is an adaptive response to the selective pressure of being abandoned by the tribe.

The most extreme kind of social rejection is that of the child by the parent, and it is believed that traditional human societies practised selective infanticide, abandonment, and other less extreme forms of reduced parental investment. Indeed, in present-day conditions of danger such as war, famine, or pestilence (ibid.), mothers invest fewer resources in their offspring, and it is this neglect and abuse rather than war itself that is the strongest depressogenic factor. Children compete with their siblings for parental resources, and one study has shown that it is the quality of childhood relationship with siblings that more strongly predicted adult depression than a bad relationship with parents. Other research showed that it was the perception of favouritism by children—favouritism in general, not towards a particular child—that predicts depression (ibid.). One adaptive theory of depression proposes that anxiety and grief (what Panksepp, 2010 calls PANIC-GRIEF) keep us close to our attachment partners, and that withdrawal and shutdown preserve energy resources and mask us from predators when abandoned by mother or mate (Watt & Panksepp, 2009).

Because humans have evolved to band together to survive, and because status—and therefore agency—within these groups determines survival, health, and acquisition of a high-quality mate, any threat to "coalitional collaboration" can be expected to increase the risk of depression. This is why the most powerful psychosocial depressogenic stimuli are social isolation, exclusion, or rejection. Stigmatisation of individuals arises because they pose a threat to the group, whether because of sickness, dependency, or cheating. It is striking that major symptoms of depression are sickness, poor self-worth, guilt, and shame, in other words an "internal state of perceived stigmatization" (Maletic & Raison, 2017, p. 103). Since depressed people have rarely done anything to warrant the feelings of worthlessness and guilt, Maletic and Raison suggest that "… abnormalities in brain systems that evolved to promote these feelings may contribute to the pathogenesis of depression" (ibid., p. 105). It turns out that depression is associated with abnormalities in structure and function in the anterior cingulate, an area that is activated in the presence of feelings of guilt or worthlessness.

One evolutionary theory posits that depression is simply an outcome of processing threats through the fight, flight, and freeze responses. In cases of chronic stress, we are repeatedly plunged into aggression, fear, or, in cases of more extreme powerlessness, immobilisation and numbness, while our positive emotions of seeking rewards and experiencing contentment are shut down (Gilbert, 2007). It is evident that all of the emotions we experience as negative (PANIC-GRIEF, FEAR, and ANGER) are nevertheless essential to our survival, and depression in its milder forms anyway helps us to survive adverse circumstances. (Other adaptive theories are outlined in Chapter 1 of this book and Chapter 5 of Dowds, 2018.)

That reproductive success (measured in terms of numbers of healthy children) is not strongly linked to depression may be explained by the nature of evolutionary strategy. It is the pursuit of pleasure that is strongly adaptive rather than reproductive success per se. (One reason for this is that reproduction in many species comes with a cost to the individual, so that natural selection competes with sexual selection.) This is why depression is associated with threats to survival and with difficulties in finding and keeping a mate rather than with having only small numbers of children (Maletic & Raison, 2017).

Social situations are the strongest drivers of mood—the integrated emotional response to our perceptions that then goes on to shape behaviour. Depressive symptoms of low mood, anxiety, reduced activity, decreased appetite, and withdrawn behaviour are advantageous in many situations that threaten our basic survival and reproductive needs. Low and anxious moods ensure that we avoid danger and maximise our resources instead of wasting time and energy on fruitless pursuits.

Psychosocial causes of depression: childhood and adult factors

The risk of major depression is increased by a wide range of factors interacting together, including: genetic liability as well as genetically influenced personality traits, poor parenting, sexual abuse and other kinds of maltreatment and traumatic experiences, loss of parent in childhood, poverty, low social support, family instability, substance abuse, and other adverse experiences throughout the lifespan (Hammen & Watkins, 2018; see Kendler et al., 2002, 2006 for references and developmental models). The environmental precursors to depression are commonly divided into two phases. In the *distal* phase, loss, stress, or trauma in childhood (including insecurely attached relationships and harsh parenting) generate vulnerability to depression. This susceptibility generally lies dormant until adolescence or adulthood when a *proximal* environmental trigger, usually further loss or stress (including an attack on one's place in the social order), exposes that vulnerability. Inevitably, there is an intergenerational component to depression whereby the consequences of stress, trauma, or loss are passed on from previous generations of a family through rearing, as well as while in the womb in the case of a stressed mother. In this chapter, I explore the consequences of our upbringing for our resilience to stress, our capacity to regulate emotions, and our ability to form relationships that combine both intimacy and autonomy.

Loss

Bowlby understood depression as frequently arising from a state of chronic, unresolved mourning, and the study of Brown and Harris (1978) showed that a majority of adverse events leading to depression entailed recent loss or expected loss: 50 per cent the loss of a close relationship (compared with 14 per cent in the non-depressed comparison group) and 20 per cent other kinds of loss (e.g. job or home). The proportion of depression that can be attributed to loss changes as other social pressures come into play. Thus, putative increases in depression in recent decades are not associated with a rise in bereavement, but with other losses (e.g. of stable communities) and stresses (e.g. changes in the environments for child rearing, and for adults an increasingly ruthless environment for work and social status).

Loss of mother during childhood was associated with an increase in the incidence of depression among adult women (Brown & Harris, 1978), and more recent research shows that the risk of depression was greater following death of the mother in childhood than after a father's demise (Hammen & Watkins, 2018). Not all children who experience loss become sensitised to depression following later losses, and the difference in outcome is associated with the type of parental care following bereavement. For example, where the child is kept in the family home, if grieving is allowed and shared, if guilt is absent, and when the surviving parent does not make strong demands for emotional support from the child, the individual can develop well despite the early loss (Bowlby, 1980).

Depressive and phobic reactions following adult bereavement depend on the circumstances surrounding the loss, in particular whether the partner's death was untimely and unexpected (Harvard study cited in Bowlby, 1980). It is the disorganisation that follows loss that, when combined with helplessness, appears to provoke depressive responses. In such a situation our interaction with the external world may be disrupted. "So long as there is active interchange between ourselves and the external world, either in thought or action, our subjective experience is not one of depression: hope, fear, anger, satisfaction, frustration, or any combination of these may be experienced. It is when interchange has ceased that depression occurs ... until such time as new patterns of interchange have become organized towards a new pattern or goal ..." (Bowlby, 1980, p. 246).

Parenting and early adversity

Retrospective studies show significant associations between depression and prior sexual or physical abuse: the more severe the abuse, the more severe and recurrent the depression. A wide range of adverse experiences, especially the cluster of "maladaptive family functioning"—a parent's mental illness, substance abuse, criminality, violence, physical and sexual abuse, and neglect—are strongly predictive of depression (Hammen & Watkins, 2018). The impact of these conditions on the children is mediated through the primary caregiver, who is usually the mother, implying that the quality of parenting is the critical factor. Indeed, prospective studies tracking the quality of parenting reliably predict adolescent and adult depression (ibid.).

Reports by depressed adults described a pattern of control (criticism, guilt induction, and intrusiveness) and an absence of affection from both parents (reviewed by Alloy et al., 2006). Of these two qualities, it was the absence of warmth and caring that had more impact on depression than the high levels of control. Observation of depressed children and adolescents also reveals difficulties in the relationship with their parents, but it can't be ruled out that the problems are generated by the depression rather than predating it. However, prospective studies confirm that an outcome of depression is associated with parental maltreatment, even after adjusting for other risk factors such as family stress or socio-economic status (Weich et al., 2009). One of the strongest risk factors for childhood-onset depression is a critical mother, and this may be one of the ways in which depressed mothers pass on the condition to their children (Gibb, 2014).

As expected, the children of harsh or uncaring parents internalise the parental criticisms into the mental states and processes typical of depression, including a sense of worthlessness and of being unlovable and incompetent augmented by constant attacks on the self. They also do not learn self-protection: how to inhibit or reinterpret psychosocial threats such as criticism or humiliating attack (Hammen & Watkins, 2018).

To sum up: critical, cold, rejecting, or over-controlling parenting lays the groundwork for vulnerability to depression at various stages in the lifespan. These are some of the causes for anxious attachment in addition to early loss or separation from caregivers, unreliable parenting, and scary, unpredictable parenting. Other early causes for depression include family disruption or stress from a wide variety of sources, which of course further reduce the parents' capacity for loving and sensitive relating.

Being victimised by other children is another consistent risk factor for childhood depression. This can take a physical form (overt victimisation) which is more common for boys, or a relational form (exclusion, spreading rumours) which is equally common among boys and girls. Prospective studies show that both kinds of bullying predict later depression (Gibb, 2014).

Neglected, abused, traumatised, and bullied children develop a heightened sensitivity to stress as a result of their early experiences. There is a direct relationship between the number of childhood adversities before the age of seventeen, and the prevalence of both MDD and PTSD following a major stressful life event in adulthood (Hammen & Watkins, 2018).

Distal and proximal factors which work together to generate depression and anxiety include: separation from or loss of attachment partners, poor affect regulation, negative models of self and other, high levels of stress, and lack of resilience to stress (of which the most potent stressor is interpersonal stress). It is readily obvious that all of these contributions including—in most cases—degrees of stress have the common underlying cause of insecure attachment. It may appear as if levels of stress are misfortunes outside the remit of the individual and this may indeed be the case in the event of natural disasters, political cataclysms such as war, or economic hardships such as inequality. However, burnout from overwork or placing the needs of the other ahead of one's own usually has elements of boosting self-esteem and proving oneself to an external or internalised other (e.g. working too hard to gain the boss's/wife's/father's approval), so the level of stress which the individual imposes on him- or herself is ultimately a consequence of insecure attachment.

Let us now explore in detail what happens in early development and how adverse experiences impact on those developmental paths.

Early development

In Toni Morrison's novel *Beloved*, a character describes what his "friend of my mind" does for him: "The pieces I am, she gather [sic] them and give them back to me in all the right order" (2007, p. 321). Winnicott (1984) intuited that we begin life as a mass of unintegrated experiences in response to novel and disconnected perceptions and stimuli. Infants rely on mother's attuned responses in order to *feel* their experience being integrated; otherwise the unintegrated material becomes dissociated. Normal dissociations include the separation of our waking from the sleeping state, or our separation from nature in urban living; but for the abused or emotionally neglected child, a great part of their waking experience remains unintegrated. For those with a childhood deficit in sensitive parenting there is an ongoing need for integration in adulthood. This was highlighted for me by a sixty-year-old depressed and anxious client who spent two years recounting her days to me just as a school child does with mother. The important thing for her was to tell me the trivial experiences of the past week with endless detail and lots of revisions to achieve greater accuracy and a fuller picture. She appeared uninterested in moving beyond this mundane narrative into issues of feeling or meaning, but seemed to regard our painstaking integration of moment by moment activities and interactions as an end in itself. Good enough mothers and therapists are friends of the mind to children and clients.

Experiencing myself as a person (what Winnicott called "personalization") arises out of repeated, consistent experiences of body-care, but it can be temporarily lost in both children and adults (1984). Depersonalisation (disembodiment) in the form of self-numbing or blanking/spacing out has a self-soothing function: we buffer ourselves as infants against stimuli for which we have no frame of reference (Eigen, 1993). When this defence becomes habitual, a chronic low-level depression ensues, as we lapse into dissociation (unintegration) where we have elements of experience that we are unable to process and organise (ibid.). This might include the pain of rejection, the terror of abandonment, the fear of censure, often because of our own unacceptable emotions, or the overwhelm of excessive stimulation—indeed anything which we feel incapable of managing.

It is important not to confuse clinical depression with Melanie Klein's depressive position, where the young child overcomes splitting as they realise that the person they love is also someone they hate. Here there is a realisation of the complexity of reality where idealisation and demonisation can no longer be mustered as reliable defences. This growing awareness is of course a bit disillusioning, but it is not usually the place of despair from which clinical depression arises. Rather, depression is "more associated with depersonalization, or hopelessness in respect of object relationships; or with a sense of futility that results from the development of a false self" (Winnicott, 1984, p. 272). It is to these emotionally absent or unattuned relationships that we now turn.

Insecure attachment

Bowlby understood clinical conditions as a disordered version of a healthy response: if the attachment figure is dangerous and unpredictable, a trusting approach is replaced with hypervigilance or withdrawal. The main source of the helplessness and hopelessness characteristic of depression is, according to Bowlby, the inability to make and maintain "affectional relationships" (1980, p. 247). In childhood, such a person may never have had a stable and secure relationship with his parents, or may have been repeatedly told that he is unlovable, inadequate, or incompetent. The quality of attachment in infancy generates working models about others in terms of their availability, trustworthiness, and ability to mentalize and respond appropriately. In the same way, the child constructs a working model of the self: her self-worth, self-awareness, and capacity for emotional self-regulation. All of these outcomes predict relationship quality and physical and psychological well-being in childhood and adulthood. Insecure attachment leads to a sense of being lonely, unlovable, and fearful of rejection, with a limited capacity to read or regulate one's own emotions or to trust, understand, or anticipate the other; it also predicts stress generation.

In later life, insecure attachment manifests within peer and romantic relationships in issues of trust, communication, ease with intimacy, and fear of abandonment (Ravitz et al., 2010). It contributes to conflict in romantic relationships, while the rejection sensitivity typical of anxious attachment predicts relationship breakdown (Hammen & Shih, 2014). The default emotions evoked by insecure attachment are sadness and fear (Dowds, 2018), so it is not surprising that the mental health difficulties associated with it are depression and anxiety in particular (Brumariu & Kearns, 2010; Hammen & Shih, 2014; Madigan et al., 2013). Loss in adulthood—whether actual or threatened—may trigger mourning and feelings of abandonment, as may be expected, but also self-criticism and a sense of helplessness and hopelessness (Hammen & Watkins, 2018).

Primary caregivers who are sensitive, responsive, and consistent generate securely attached children, whereas those who are unavailable, dismissive, or hostile towards the child's emotions raise an insecure avoidant child. Those who are inconsistently available raise an insecure ambivalent (anxiously attached) child and those who are terrifying or terrified give rise to disorganised attachment in the child. Interaction with insensitive, inconsistent, or terrifying attachment figures in childhood interferes with the development of a secure, stable sense of self, reduces resilience to stress, and predisposes the individual to break down in times of challenge or crisis. Hundreds of studies (cross-sectional, longitudinal, and prospective) show that insecure attachment (of all kinds) correlates with a wide range of mental disorders including depression, generalised anxiety disorder (GAD), OCD, PTSD, personality disorders, and schizophrenia (Mikulincer & Shaver, 2007, 2013). Likewise, insecure attachment plays a role in predicting postpartum depression (Ikeda et al., 2014).

Attachment insecurity is not in itself sufficient to generate mental disorders. Rather it interacts with genetic endowment, temperament, intelligence, and life history, including abuse, to pave the way for major depression (Mikulincer & Shaver, 2007, 2013). For example, many studies reveal no link between avoidant attachment and generalised distress, but for subjects exposed to highly stressful events there is an association.

Similarly, abuse in childhood (physical, psychological, or sexual) inter-acts with insecure attachment to increase the frequency of depression in adults compared with either vulnerability factor acting alone. Stressful life events or threats to well-being (poverty, physical health problems, turbulent romantic relationships) strengthen the association between insecure attachment and psychopathology. More longitudinal studies are needed to reveal the details of how other factors such as family adversity or genetics may modify the link between insecure attachment and depression.

A complication in interpreting correlations is that insecure attach-ment creates vulnerability to psychopathology, but psychopathology can also deepen attachment insecurity. For example, a prior history of depression or abuse increased the likelihood of women's attachment insecurity worsening after the stress and loss of an abortion (Mikulincer & Shaver, 2013). Indeed, one of the symptoms of depression is with-drawal from human contact and/or increased neediness for help or reas-surance, which have a systemic impact on the attachment partner and hence on the depressed individual (Coyne, 1985).

Attachment orientation and emotional regulation

Insecure attachment leads to fragmentation of the self, lack of internal coherence, and unstable self-esteem overly dependent on the approval of others. Insecure people are prone to defences like perfectionism to counter feelings of worthlessness, as well as narcissism to inflate self-esteem. People with an avoidant style are more prone to grandiosity (overt narcissism), while those with an ambivalent style tend to be self-obsessed and hypersensitive to other people's evaluation of them (covert narcissism) (Mikulincer & Shaver, 2013).

In healthy development, "… the environment [including the other] is discovered without loss of sense of self" (Winnicott, 1984, p. 222). On the other hand, in the face of ongoing misattunement, the child cannot but react to the impingement and lose their sense of self, which is "only regained by a return to isolation" (ibid.). Coming to associate contact with others with loss of self leads to introversion at the least, or in more extreme cases to depression, where the individual has given up all hope for meaningful relationships. It is very important to understand this in working with depressed clients, not just in terms of the necessity for attunement, but also in terms of attempting to ameliorate their tendency to self-isolate only gradually. Many texts on depression regard isolating in very negative terms, and of course in the long run it can only exacerbate depression. However, as Winnicott realised, temporary withdrawal to shield a fragile and damaged sense of self is essential in the short term before the work of building the self can progress.

Emotional dysregulation mediates the link between attachment insecurity and psychopathology. Securely attached people are more aware of their emotions and have more constructive strategies for regulating them, such as problem solving, reappraisal, and support seeking. The insecurely attached, on the other hand, have serious difficulties in identifying, describing, and regulating emotions. Problems in regulating emotions also mediate their difficulties in being mindfully present in the here and now (Mikulincer & Shaver, 2019). Depression and anxiety are characterised, not just by a high frequency of negative emotions, but also by the individual interpreting and responding to the emotions in a negative feedback loop. Cognitive patterns such as catastrophising, becoming phobic about emotions, believing that the low mood will last forever, believing that they cannot change, having little tolerance for uncertainty—all contribute not only to feeling low, but also to a stuck mood.

Avoidants inhibit emotions and leave distress unacknowledged and unresolved (deactivation strategy). This generates the rigid stuck mood characteristic of depression, and to the phenomenon that avoidants can be cold, introverted, or competitive in relationship. When exposed to chronic, uncontrollable, severely distressing events, or conditions of high cognitive load, they become overwhelmed by their hitherto suppressed emotions.

Ambivalents, on the other hand, tend to amplify their feelings and exaggerate their problems (hyperactivation) because this strategy sometimes attracts intimacy and care. But in the long term, hyperactivation of emotions generates patterns of anxiety and panic, which become habitual and difficult to shift. Furthermore, the hysterical, impulsive demands on others, sometimes including outbursts of anger or violence (Mikulincer & Shaver, 2013, 2019), tend to alienate partners and friends.

Perceived problems with regulating emotions were found to mediate the association of insecure attachment with both depression and GAD; while not accepting negative emotions, and being unable to control impulsive behaviours, was the mediating form of emotional dysregulation in the case of GAD (Marganska, 2013). In addition, maladaptive perfectionism mediated the relationship between avoidant and ambivalent attachment styles and depression, hopelessness, and life satisfaction; while adaptive perfectionism formed a bridge between avoidant attachment and hopelessness and life satisfaction (Gnilka et al., 2013).

Anxiety

Our helplessness in infancy is reason enough for anxiety, but good enough parents shield the child from an awareness of its helplessness by fostering an illusion of omnipotence (Winnicott, 1990). It is when that adaptation and attunement fail badly that we begin to feel chronic anxiety. Separation anxiety inevitably accompanies insecure attachment, whether explicitly experienced by those with ambivalent or disorganised attachment, or defended against but lying in wait for a trigger to release it as in avoidant attachment. Losses of loved ones in adulthood, or losses of job, home, country, or other elements of the environment that contribute to security and identity can all provoke acute anxiety and attachment-related depression.

Anxiety is of course an essential emotion in warning us of potential danger, and indeed hypophobic people get into trouble or have shorter lives (Lee et al., 2006). Dysfunctional anxiety, on the other hand (Barlow et al., 2014), is characterised by a greater frequency and intensity of the feeling; less clarity about its causes; excessive vigilance and intolerance for uncertainty or ambivalence; defences of avoidance and suppression; and the resultant amplification of the fear of fear. The last features can't be emphasised enough. It is *how* we relate to and process anxiety or low mood that is crucial in both generating and recovering from mood disorders.

Attunement and the depressed dyad

Secure attachment generates self-awareness, emotional regulation, the capacity to mentalize others, resilience to stress, and good mental and physical health. The fortunate infant whose primary caregiver is sensitive, perceptive, responsive, and predictable is likely to be securely attached and resilient in the face of stress or loss in later life (Siegel, 2012). For example, bereavement is met with grief but, with time, the individual can reorganise themselves and generate a satisfying way of living in the absence of the loved one. For the insecurely attached adult, however, the response to bereavement and other threats to security, blows to self-worth, or stressful demands can shatter rigid defences, expose the fragile sense of self, and lead to a depressive breakdown. What these insecurely attached people have lacked in childhood is an unthreatening, reliable source of sensitive attunement which calms the infant in the face of stress, and which can read their moment-by-moment changing needs. Attunement is particularly inadequate in the case of depressed caregivers, and about 40 per cent of the offspring of depressed mothers experience depression themselves by the age of sixteen (Gerhardt, 2015).

We will now examine how infants adapt to a depressed mother in such a way that they develop a long-term propensity to depression. In the case of good enough parenting the child finds *himself* in the mother's facial response to his overtures (Winnicott, 1990), but the depressed mother is unable to respond sensitively to the child and may react to the child's cries of hunger or pain with numbness, impatience, or rage. In the face of such ongoing misattunement, the child experiences shame and humiliation (Schore, 1996). Eventually the child learns to adapt to the mother's needs in a reversal of the good enough state of affairs. They learn to quell their own needs, including their vitality, and learn to disconnect the developing psyche from the demands or feedback from the soma.

Depressed people swing back and forth between the anger, agitation, and anxiety of the SNS and the shutdown of the dorsal vagus as we saw in Chapter 3. The children of a depressed mother typically experience her as angry, rough, and intrusive, interspersed with being blanked out and absent (Gerhardt, 2015; Siegel, 2012). This absence of "maternal presence, engagement and vitality may all be experienced as life threatening" (Cozolino, 2010, p. 268). The switched off state feels a greater threat than mother's hostility because we (even as adults) lose the sense of existing when faced with a relational void (see Tronick et al., 1978 for the still-face experiment). Infants develop emotional complexity and a sense of meaning by knowing how they feel about interpersonal experiences. In order to process and organise this new information they need psycho-feedback from the mother, who shows them who they are, who she is, and what to expect from relationships. However, when the mother is depressed and the child adapts by being sad with her, he develops coherence (self-organisation) and complexity only in the short term (Tronick & Beeghly, 2011). Over time the child's self-organisation becomes constricted and rigid, and he fails to acquire flexibility, vitality, complexity, and coherence (Siegel, 2012). When grown up, this individual often has the depressive's combination of low mood and stuck mood, where thoughts, feelings, memories, and perceptions are skewed towards a rigid, anxious down state.

Stern (2000) distinguishes categorical affects such as sadness, fear, anger, etc. from vitality affects which refer to the kinetics of arousal such as surging, fleeting, drawn out, etc. He illustrates the distinction with the example of puppets who cannot express categorical affects because of the absence of facial expression. But their vitality affects reveal who they are through the drooping limbs and head of the lethargic character, or the jaunty bounce of a cheerful one. It is thought that infants initially perceive vitality affects rather than discrete acts such as mother reaching for the bottle. In the case of the depressed individual these vitality affects are less fluid, so that feelings of sadness or anxiety become solidified into fixed *states* of depression.

Depressed mothers cannot comfort or soothe their children out of negative feelings, with the result that the child learns the pattern of ruminating on how bad, unlovable, or incompetent he is. Such children then find it hard to learn how to solve problems or distract themselves from painful feelings. Likewise, depressed mothers are much less likely to repair ruptures in attunement—indeed the relationship is one long history of misattunement. These children become adults who resolve interpersonal conflict by attack or withdrawal (fight or flight). This is quite distinct from the trusting, mentalizing *engagement* of the ventral vagus, where the securely attached can make a stab at what is going on for the other, trust her to mentalize adequately, and forgive themselves and the other for their mentalizing deficits.

Depression and deficits of the self

Relational failures result in a variety of different forms of non-resilient self, collectively known as fragile self (Dowds, 2018). A resilient sense of self has the properties of cohesion, vitality, and harmony (Kohut & Wolf, 1986); affect and body regulation, intuition, empathy, attuned communication, and response flexibility (Siegel, 2010); as well as autonomy and the capacity to meet one's own needs and to love others (Miller, 1986).

Alice Miller has pointed out that: "Depression can be understood as a sign of the loss of self and consists of a denial of one's emotional reactions and feelings. This denial begins in the service of an absolutely essential adaptation during childhood, to avoid losing the object's love" (1986, p. 334). Pathological self formation thus originates in childhood strategies to maintain at all costs the attachment bond, however non-facilitative. Different deficits of self underlie or trigger depression in different ways: depression can be a reaction to a fragmented self because of unresolved inner conflicts; or to a false self because the individual is cut off from his organismic needs.

The defences against depression lead to problems of their own. The inflation of narcissists is a defence against the inherent depression associated with an empty sense of self. Other overcompensations for a fragile self include: manic activity which can result in burnout (see Dowds, 2018 for examples); or mindless obsessional repetition as evoked so poignantly by Guntrip. "The experience of doing in the absence of a secure sense of being degenerates into a meaningless succession of mere activities (as in the obsessional's meaningless repetition of the same thought, word or act), not performed for their own proper purpose but as a futile effort to 'keep oneself in being', to manufacture a sense of 'being' one does not possess" (Guntrip, 1992, p. 254).

For a much longer discussion on this topic, see Chapter 8 of Dowds (2018).

Intergenerational transmission

Depression is transmitted from one generation to another, not just through the genes, but also through the maternal rearing environment exerting emotional, cognitive, and behavioural effects. Attachment patterns are passed on through the generations (Cozolino, 2010; Gerhardt, 2015). In the absence of therapeutic intervention, an individual is likely to parent their children in the same way as they were parented. Emotions will be regulated, exaggerated, or repressed in the same manner.

For example, an atmosphere of anxiety as well as defences against it (e.g. hyperactivity leading to burnout) are conveyed to offspring. A sense of the world as being unsafe, and of the individual being unable to deal with it is passed on from overprotective parents. Behaviour in relationships will be replicated in an interdependent, distancing, or pursuing manner; power may be distributed between peers, or divided according to bully and victim.

Most strikingly, the impact of stress and trauma is passed on, even to descendants who have not been told about the trauma of their ancestors (see Dowds, 2018 for examples), as each generation of parent, not having been soothed themselves, cannot comfort and calm their own children. A mother who is traumatised transmits her own dysregulated affect to her offspring. Doubt has been cast on whether epigenetic markers can be transmitted in the germ line (see Chapter 2), but it is certainly the case that a stressed pregnant woman can pass stress on to her offspring: by cortisol crossing the placenta (Di Pietro et al., 2006), and by the foetal DNA being epigenetically modified in response to maternal stress (Roth & Sweatt, 2011; Yehuda et al., 2005; plus Chapter 2 above).

Adult triggers: inauthenticity and damaging relationships

See Dowds (2018) for a much more detailed discussion of the material covered in the remainder of this chapter.

Insecure attachment and loss or stress in infancy generate a weak or fragmented sense of self. This shaky foundation affects our resilience to stress and loss and our capacity to form and maintain stable and meaningful relationships in adulthood. In the absence of psychotherapy, we usually replicate the attachment pattern with parents in the way we relate to partners, spouses, and children in later life. Thus, we have the same dysregulation of emotions, a similar miscommunication and instability in relationship, and a poor capacity to regulate stress through relationship (co-regulation). Having a weak sense of self, we may lapse into depression and anxiety in adolescence. Alternatively, having an external locus of evaluation, we may compensate for poor self-esteem or a sense of inner emptiness by overworking or otherwise trying to be extra good, nice, or competent, or to appear independent, successful, or powerful. This eventually leads to burnout because we are not motivated by our own authentic drives, beliefs, or needs, but are driven by what is supposedly valued by other individuals (e.g. parents) or society at large (e.g. the denizens of social media). Such a false sense of self is inherently depressogenic as well as generating heavy loads of stress, and it can be difficult to access true self impulses because of the poor psycho-feedback such individuals have received in childhood. They are out of touch with their needs and emotions: they may not recognise when they feel phony, threatened, or exhausted and have no idea how to feel real, or what it would entail to have an internal locus of evaluation.

Theorists of human needs have agreed that we have innate and non-negotiable psychosocial needs: for security, competence, connection, autonomy, and authenticity (Kasser, 2002; Maslow, 1943). Fromm (1990) emphasised the human-specific needs that arise from our consciousness of our separateness from ourselves, other people, nature, and the world. These needs are for: relationships, human roots, identity, a frame of orientation and devotion, and ways to transcend our powerlessness. Many people prone to depression are unaware of their need for or how to achieve an authentic autonomous identity (true self), as we have noted. In addition, they are often well aware of their loneliness, but have no idea how to engage in relationships in a way that would add to rather than subtract from their sense of self. This is because the caregiving they received as children was insensitive and/or aggressive so that they *expect* misunderstanding, judgement, exclusion, manipulation, or abuse. These individuals then become isolated, despite often being surrounded by people. Humans have a lifelong need for the positive but accurate mirroring that tells us who we are and makes us feel acceptable (Lessem, 2005). We need intimate relationships not just for initial development but also for maintenance of the self, for meaning, and for feeling safe. We also need a broader connection to a community to acquire an extended sense of self as part of something larger. For many prone to depression, they are in a double bind with respect to relationships: they lose self within them and lose self without them. The good news is that psychotherapy that foregrounds the relationship can help a client identify and overcome their particular relational traps: for example, passively yielding power to others; not knowing what is real or meaningful when a powerful other negates their sense of reality; introjecting the projections of others; believing others' harsh judgements; accepting unfair accusations; placing the other ahead of oneself—and many other variations of emotional incompetence and lack of boundaries against impingement, entanglement, and abuse.

A further complication of underlying depression is that people distract themselves from it with a range of addictions—to alcohol, drugs, eating, sex, risk, shopping, wealth accumulation, or ceaseless activity including workaholism. These defences deepen the depression, either physiologically in the case of alcohol and some drugs, or with the gradual realisation of how empty and meaningless these pursuits are. Many people have depressive breakdowns when they collapse at the end of a very busy, stressful period, which in some cases includes having reached the pinnacle of long-sought success (Dowds, 2018).

To sum up, adult triggers of depression can be stress (e.g. from overwork, poverty, stressful social relationships) or loss (e.g. through divorce, loss of home, job, community, health, a beloved natural environment), usually because of how these directly or indirectly interact with already poor relationships and a weak sense of self. Most stress is social (e.g. he can't stand up to the boss; she feels unpopular in her peer group) and results in humiliation, exclusion, helplessness, or hopelessness: signs of low social status or exclusion from the social order.

While an initial episode of depression is usually provoked by negative life events, the depressed person can then contribute to generating further negative events, thus setting in train a vicious cycle of stress generation. In addition, cognitive biases can moderate or amplify the impact of life stresses, and depressed people tend to have attributional and inferential styles that reinforce or fail to buffer negative events (Gibb, 2014), for instance feeling guilty for letting other people down because you have not followed the path they have laid out for your life; blaming yourself for being bullied, etc.

Social influences and increases in depression

Because our genes evolve far too slowly to have played any role, the apparent increase in depression in recent years must derive from changes in how we are living. Some of these changes affect how children develop so that they are more prone to depression; while some affect triggers in adulthood (Dowds, 2018).

Deregulation of capitalism, globalisation, climate change, and breakdown in extended and nuclear families have drastically changed the social world and therefore the world in which the self is shaped and maintained. Social cohesion and trust in each other or in our politicians or other authority figures have declined. The increased wealth gap within and between countries and between generations, the growth of the "precariat", and the fluidity of the workplace (London today, Bangalore tomorrow) have decimated communities, generated a huge underclass and millions of economic refugees, and institutionalised social and economic instability. We are now far more likely to live lonely, isolated lives without a stable or trusted community and often without a family. One outcome of the changes in the economy is that young children grow up in an environment where both parents have to work, so infants develop without the co-regulated emotional interactions that generate secure attachment (Gerhardt, 2011). Insecure (particularly avoidant) attachment is on the rise, along with individualism, narcissism, and materialism (Twenge, 2014). Our relationships are now less characterised by trust and cooperation and more by competitive individualism where the other is a rival or evaluator or both. Relationships have been contaminated by consumerist ideology: on dating sites, for example, people advertise their brand, and the buyer hesitates in choosing for fear of missing out on a better bargain somewhere else in the apparently limitless virtual marketplace.

A separate problem that has enabled and become intertwined with neoliberal capitalism arises from the hyper-connectedness of information technology. Far from solving the problem of loneliness, the supposed connection of online contact both leaves us with a shadow of the richness of face-to-face relationships, and directly impacts on the nature of the self. We are now lonelier than ever before, a trend that has been greatly exacerbated by the take-up of social media (Murphy, 2020). Multiple studies have found an association between social media use and depression, anxiety, self-esteem, and sleep quality (e.g. Cleland Woods & Scott, 2016; Lin et al., 2016).

Some of the adverse psychological impacts of mobile phones, social media, and IT in general are listed below:

- Demand for immediate answers: the overload and immediacy of emails are a major source of workplace stress (e.g. Brown et al., 2014).
- Loss of desire or ability to relate to other human beings (including failure to learn how to cope with conflict) because of addiction to screens. Most damagingly, this includes a decline in parents engaging

face to face with their offspring so that some children now have to be taught at school how to read the human face (Rowson & McGilchrist, 2017).

- No down-time to engage the restorative default neurological network—which is detrimental to well-being and to attention to others.
- Fragmented attention.
- Drop in attention span from twelve to eight seconds in a decade, according to a Microsoft study.
- More attention is hived off into dealing with technological problems than ever before, generating more and more left-brain dominance at the expense of the meaning-generating right hemisphere (Dowds, 2021; McGilchrist, 2010).
- Sex "education" through online pornography is leading boys to believe that abuse of girls is normal sexual activity.
- Normalisation and expression of hatred of all except the in-group.
- Undermining of democracy.
- Work outsourced to the consumer for which we are untrained and for which the promised "help lines" serve only to frustrate ("try our website") and emphasise that you are on your own in solving problems (called "shadow work" by Ivan Illich).
- Social media generate the greatest problems for the self: loss of privacy; impoverishment of inner experiencing; external locus of evaluation; addiction to performance and ego rewards; loneliness because of loss of face-to-face contact. Even the small proportion of the population that doesn't engage with social media are affected by it because not listening, dissembling, boasting, making choices based on what will look/sound good have become the accepted mode of social discourse. Most worryingly, the erosion of authentic identity in adults affects their capacity to parent the next generation.
- One combined effect of neoliberal capitalism and social media is the erosion of trust. The other has become a competitor or evaluator or both (Verhaeghe, 2014). As we become hyper-individualised, society becomes atomised. It is a moot point which of these outcomes is more destructive.

These are just some of the problems arising from the revolution in information technology. As a therapist I see its strongest impact on young women struggling with anxiety and depression. They are disembodied, have an arid inner life, little sense of what being authentic would mean, and their defining motivation is to impress or at least keep up with their peer group.

We are living at a time where the natural world is being destroyed through population growth, pollution, and global warming, we are losing cohesive human communities and trust in our fellow human beings, and we are replacing the richness of the self with the poverty of a grasping, addictive, performing ego. All true connection—to self, others, and the world—is thereby being eroded. Connection—however demanding and difficult it can sometimes be with our fellow humans—is what gives our lives meaning, and in its absence we sink into despair and depression, or hatred and rage.

Conclusions

The foundations of depression are laid down in adverse experiences in childhood, particularly circumstances that affect the capacity of the primary carer to parent her child in a loving, attuned manner. Abuse (including harsh criticism), rejection, loss, neglect, trauma, addiction, family instability, and other upheavals all contribute to the child being blocked from developing the strong and resilient sense of self that comes from emotional regulation within securely attached relationships. As such children grow up, the fragile sense of self with its allied defences proves to be inadequate for the more complex relational world of adulthood. For example, they may feel so powerless in relationships that they are repeatedly victimised and bullied, or they may burn out through overcompensating for poor self-esteem. They will be unable to achieve the balance between autonomy and intimacy that characterises adult relationships capable of sustaining and co-regulating us. These individuals are vulnerable to stress, loneliness, depression, and anxiety, so that setbacks that other people might override reignite their childhood experiences: for instance, a relatively minor social embarrassment may trigger the old humiliations from the past along with the self-hatred which is always waiting in the wings.

We are moving into an increasingly unstable, unequal, impinging society dominated by competitive individualism. Family and community breakdown in particular threaten our security, identity, connection, and source of meaning, and face-to-face relationships are being replaced by performances for social media. People with childhood and/or genetic vulnerability are less able to withstand the ruthlessness, loneliness, alienation, and sensory overload that characterise twenty-first-century urban life, but they affect us all.

Part II

Psychotherapy: mobilisation and meaning

Depression is difficult to treat. By its nature, it is a stuck and inflexible condition. It is a disorder of the self and of relationships and is also an intensely embodied state. Therapy must engage with all aspects of depression and not treat it as merely a mental, or a purely intrapsychic process. The initial focus often needs to be on helping the client find sufficient hope and trust to keep attending. The ideas in this section of the book should not be treated as a recipe. Like all clients, depressed people need above all to be *heard* by the therapist, and to begin to hear themselves. Any technique used must be a response to an active call—whether explicit or implicit—from the client. The discussion that follows makes suggestions about how to engage with particularly demanding aspects of the state that arise from the very object relations that have created it in the first place.

Depression is commonly characterised as an absence of aliveness, but the solution is not simply to try to increase vitality directly. This is because depression is at the same time a *defence* against aliveness, so therapy must first increase tolerance of affect. Rapid shattering of the defence—even if this were possible—would uncover torrents of grief, anxiety, terror, rage, or simply vitality that have not been accepted or regulated, and are therefore likely to be experienced as overwhelming and unmanageable.

My approach is informed by psychodynamic developmental theory as well as knowledge from the biosciences, and it is rooted in a humanistic understanding of the nature of the therapeutic relationship. In short it incorporates psychodynamic content into a humanistic practice. This involves—as appropriate—elements of person-centred therapy, Gestalt, creative arts, and body psychotherapies. The aim is the client's growth towards an autonomous, authentic, and embodied self, capable of both independence and intimacy in relationships. In many cases the work must range between a focus on the client's characteristic pattern of threat responses to work on awareness of triggers, body responses, and the discovery of alternative modes of relating. The orientation is as much towards the present as the past. Because respect, trust, and grounded reality are viewed as critical in the therapeutic relationship, the client's responses are not treated as delusional or entirely a consequence of their parental relationships. Instead they are understood as reactions which were valid and creative in childhood, but may not currently be applicable all the time, so that a very gradual shift can occur in the way in which the client relates to self and other.

Chapter 5 examines what the depression may be telling the client, and provides inspiration from other sufferers who have transformed their lives by listening to the message about their way of living that is held within their low mood. In Chapter 6 I suggest some ways in which the therapist can find the parts of the client that are not stuck and that want change. Chapter 7 explores ways of working with key aspects of depression: attachment, the fragile self, the polyvagal system, all of which of course are intimately intertwined, as well as specific issues that are not always present, including anxiety and bereavement. Chapter 8 presents a case study of a client who, despite holding down a job, nevertheless displayed the symptoms of anhedonia, self-loathing, exhaustion, and a sense of hopelessness and futility. I explore the progress of the three years of therapy we did together.

CHAPTER 5

The message from within: moving towards authenticity

Macbeth:

Canst thou not minister to a mind diseased,
Pluck from the memory a rooted sorrow,
Raze out the written troubles of the brain,
And with some sweet oblivious antidote
Cleanse the stuffed bosom of that perilous stuff
Which weighs upon the heart?

Doctor:

Therein the patient must minister to himself.

—*Macbeth*, Act V Scene iii

No man hath affliction enough, that is not matured and ripened by it,
and made fit for God by that affliction.

—John Donne, *Devotions upon Emergent Occasions,*
Meditation 17

One of the social trends that is partly responsible for the increased incidence of depression is at the same time a considerable block against a
client engaging in psychotherapy. This is the tendency to instrumentalise

the self which is amplified by our current hyper-competitive culture of performance and winning. As a result, many people view depression as a "disease" in which the brain is a broken machine that needs fixing. This is the technological/medical model of depression: within this way of thinking, illness has no meaning or message for us, and suffering is therefore pointless rather than the opportunity for the ripening that Donne envisaged. Seeing oneself in mechanistic terms, and evaluated by one's capacity to perform, constitutes a world view that drains meaning from life (Dowds, 2021) and actually contributes to depression. Implicit in this view are the beliefs that (a) there is something defective in me; (b) depression is a fixed *condition* rather than a mutable *process*, an interactive engagement with life. Clients who instrumentalise themselves typically have a life plan that is being frustrated or delayed by this inconvenient malfunctioning and frequently see depression as a weakness and therefore the sign of a "loser". If instead we see anxiety and depression as about a fragmented self, insecure attachment, emotional baggage from the past along with limiting and outdated beliefs about yourself and the world, these moods convey a message which must be addressed. Depression is no different from any other prolonged emotion: moods are signals that inform us whether we experience the environment as safe, welcoming, stimulating, calming, nurturing, empowering, meaningful—or not—and therefore whether we withdraw or engage joyfully. And we can listen and respond appropriately as we would with other emotions. The medical profession and CBT treat negative feelings as undesirable but essentially meaningless epiphenomena of depression; but as the psychoanalyst Mark Solms has argued trenchantly, feelings are telling us something and there is a good reason why depression feels bad (Solms, 2012; Solms & Panksepp, 2010).

Taking responsibility for your own recovery

In my previous book (Dowds, 2018), I used published memoirs of depressive breakdown to provide an experiential account of what this process feels like. Here I will allude again to these writings to reveal how individuals can either learn or fail to engage with what their depression has to teach them. The crucial factor in recovering from depression is to take responsibility for the condition. This is not about self-blame, but about reaching a deep understanding of the psychodynamic genesis of the process so that you can move beyond it. In Daphne Merkin's article about psychotherapy (2010), she doesn't give a head count but mentions thirteen different therapists—mostly or all psychoanalysts and with the title of Dr—who she saw over a forty-year period. She is constantly on a quest for a therapist who could make her happy, but despite her extensive experience, she isn't sure that she has much greater self-knowledge than other people. Merkin appears not to have made the shift from expecting the therapist to rescue her to the knowledge that, as the Doctor says in *Macbeth*, she has to transform herself: "I failed to grasp that there was no magic to be had, that a therapist's insights weren't worth anything unless you made them your own and that nothing that had happened to me already could be undone, no matter how many times I went over it." Did therapy infantalise her so that she was unable to move into the more empowered position of taking responsibility for her own life? I have to wonder whether she might not have been much better served by a humanistic therapist, who would have made it clear that she needed to reach her own insights and would have actively engaged with her in an authentic healing relationship. Merkin ends the article by freeing herself from one therapist without having another lined up. Yet, she felt sure that little time would pass before she started off again.

An essential prerequisite for psychotherapy is faith that, as Eigen says, "emotional truth is possible" (1993, p. 124). This means accepting that there is a difference between authentic, organismic drives (true self) and beliefs and behaviour that are socially adaptive, but individually inauthentic (false self). Part and parcel of this is belief in process and the possibility of change from an external to an internal locus of evaluation. It entails being willing to be flexible about goals and standards, to follow authentic impulses rather than the dictates of the will. My client Shelley (Dowds, 2018) described herself and her family members in terms set in stone, and such a belief that emotion is fixed rather than malleable leads to higher rates of depression, less reappraisal of situations, and poorer social adjustment (Tamir et al., 2007). This and other belief systems that block recovery must be challenged as they emerge in therapy. But rather than attacking them, the depth therapist investigates their meaning or function. In Shelley's case, her rigid view of her personality arose from her clinging to any identity, however thin or negative, in order simply to have an identity. This, of course, made the work very slow, because if she was to gain a larger and more authentic sense of self, she had to give up the illusion of identity that had been her lifebelt. Shelley was equally insistent that nothing in the circumstances of her life would change. When, despite herself, things—relationships, job, our relationship in her therapy—did change and improve, Shelley sabotaged them. She had such a dread that happiness would be stolen from her—as she felt it was after the family moved from a working-class to a middle-class district when she was twelve—that it was preferable to maintain her depressed state than to risk hope being dashed and paradise being lost again.

Taking charge of one's recovery requires trust in one's capacity to develop awareness, to learn, and to transform. Such trust is difficult for people who have no interest in their inner process or who have an unshakable belief that the way they are is immutable. They may not wish to take responsibility for their depression and rely instead on conventional medical-model treatments, like antidepressants and CBT. Such suppressive techniques may ameliorate the symptoms—temporarily at least—if for instance you are one of the lucky one-third or so of the population who respond well to antidepressant drugs. However, they will not help you learn the *meaning* of your depression, why it manifested in the first place. As one person who has listened and responded to her depression says: "If you agree to demonize depression, you won't be able to truly alleviate it, no matter what you do. You'll have few skills, impaired emotional agility, and no true grasp of what is occurring in your psyche or your world" (McLaren, 2015, p. 30). The passive and the indolent—and it is admittedly hard not to be like this when depressed—may hope that love will heal them. But as James Gordon, a professor of mind–body medicine cautions: "The love of others cannot ultimately sustain us. If we haven't changed what made us depressed—the imbalances and distortions that our demons cause, the unmet needs and unfulfilled potential—we will eventually drain the other's love of its healing force and warp it to fit our still-crippled form" (Gordon, 2015). One reason why love on its own cannot be a remedy is that, if we have attachment difficulties, sooner or later even an initially positive relationship will evoke dysregulation as our earlier patterns are activated.

Those who fail to learn awareness keep relapsing until they find out what their depression is about. Mark Rice-Oxley, whose depression seems to have been triggered by stress, returned to work after a relapse and wrote an article on depression for *The Guardian*. It was reprinted in the *Daily Mail* and received a huge response. He relapsed again. In the meantime, Dorothy Rowe responded to his article in her blog, saying: "The chances are that he will become depressed again until … he learns the lesson that his depression can teach him" (Rice-Oxley, 2012, p. 260). I had the same response to his account. Rice-Oxley took his medication unquestioningly but gives no feedback on whether it worked. He faithfully followed his CBT regime and did his homework. He tracked down his patterns from the outside, but didn't explore his inner process, make discoveries for himself, or engage with himself emotionally. This may be partly his own mind-blindness, but the CBT approach can't have helped him get beyond it. By his lights he did his best, but he really doesn't get what the therapy process should/could be about. When asked about his overall life meaning or purpose he was blank. Like many in the twenty-first century, he has no framework round which to build meaning; he replaces meaning with doing his best at each individual task he performs. The existential therapist Emmy van Deurzen-Smith (1997) shows how we can gain meaning from each of the four dimensions of living: the physical, social, psychological, and spiritual. From these, we can gain meaning through efficacy, relationships, identity, and connection respectively (see also Dowds, 2018). A relatively low-level satisfaction can be found in efficacy, but this does not come close to what can be obtained in the social or psychological dimensions, much less the ultimate meaning of the spiritual plane. But Rice-Oxley did learn a lesson about acceptance—about the fact that a process deeper than his will was in charge. As he says: "Recovery is another of those diabolical passive verbs. You don't recover from depression: recovery comes to find you. When it's good and ready" (2012, p. 299).

While Rice-Oxley appeared to take responsibility for his recovery, in fact he was too obedient in adhering to what the experts told him to do, rather than what his embodied self was telling him. Both he and Merkin—at the time of their respective writings—could have benefitted from a greater awareness, which can come about only by being less dependent and compliant. Andrew Solomon (2014), on the other hand, had the awareness, but chose to remain dependent on medication because he didn't want to change his lifestyle.

The American journalist Tracy Thompson (1995) eventually did take responsibility for her recovery and came to understand her depression as resulting from emotional dishonesty. While on suicide watch in hospital, she was resistant to and cynical about group therapy and the various movement and relaxation exercises provided, so she decided to fake her way into discharge. In the face of humiliating feedback from the other patients, she began to challenge her various forms of dishonesty: lying, denial, selective amnesia, etc. She came to realise how these forms of emotional dishonesty allowed her to remain a victim, and she started to change—initially, it is true, just to avoid being criticised by her fellow inmates. She then became aware of some of her own emotional patterns through seeing them in other patients—such as her phoniness and inability to connect. Various cases she covered as a legal affairs reporter, where criminals pleaded diminished responsibility, caused her to question whether she herself took responsibility for her actions. She began to give herself credit for achievements and to stay with her anxiety. She struggled with moving from an external to an internal locus of self-esteem because of the danger of fooling herself: "What if you *think* you're terrific, but you're really an asshole?" (1995, p. 273). Finally, she realised that we need both to love ourselves and to be open—in a self-forgiving way—to being judged by others. Thompson *did* have to learn to love herself, but also to be honestly tough with herself. However, her self-awareness didn't go beyond owning up to her cognitive and behavioural patterns: she still saw herself from an external locus and didn't appear to get in touch with the needs and drives of her organismic/authentic self.

Learning from depression

I want to repeat that recovery from depression requires a philosophical shift away from seeing depression as a genetic or brain disease. Insofar as there is an intrinsic vulnerability—for example, through gene variants or because a stressful infancy programmed a heightened HPA response—the way in which that vulnerability manifests is clearly contextual and dependent on how it interacts with our current way of living. In order to be open to transformation, clients and therapists need to view depression as an adaptive response to formative circumstances, past and present. Jung regarded depression as an unconscious compensation: to find its meaning, an awakening process of descent and initiation were necessary. "This can only be done by consciously regressing along with the depressive tendency and integrating the memories so activated in the conscious mind—which is what the depression was aiming at in the first place" (Jung, 1956, p. 404). We must stop seeing depression as a problem to be fixed, but rather as a message from the unconscious urgently demanding our attention. As Joseph Campbell observed: "It is only by going down into the abyss that we recover the treasures of life. Where you stumble, there lies your treasure" (1949, p. 85). The key questions are: "What is my depression telling me and what is it asking of me?" This will usually be a combination of the need to acknowledge and heal past wounds, while at the same time changing the current self-destructive way of living which is often a crumbling defence against a fragile sense of self. Depression is an opportunity for rebirth—like the sun, which "sails over the sea like an immortal god who every evening is immersed in the maternal waters and is born anew in the morning" (Jung, 1956, p. 209).

This resonant image implies trust, as I have said in my previous book:

> Taking personal responsibility and trusting their process is easier for those who can re-vision and hold the depression in a more expansive, quasi-spiritual framework, though this need not always involve a formal spiritual practice. Exemplars of such trust are to be found in the contributors to *Darkness Before Dawn*, a collection of short personal accounts by spiritually-minded people who have suffered from depression (edited by Simon, 2015). One saw that despair cracked open her heart (Pipher); another understood that depression was a friend (Palmer); or "a pain that's a solution to a deeper pain" (Masters); others experienced it as "ingenious stagnation" (McLaren); "initiation" (Roberts, Ingerman); or "a wake-up call" (Foster). As Michael Beckwith (2015, p. 73) observes in the same volume: "Every moment of seeming self-disintegration is, in truth, a reintegration of the self with the Self", which succinctly captures the movement into expansion. (Dowds, 2018, p. 259)

For the most detailed account of getting under the skin of her depression, we must go to a poet and Buddhist practitioner. Gwyneth Lewis viewed the period of her depression as "a dark room where you're developing the next chapter of your life before living it" (2002, p. 96). She learned that her depression arose from overriding her real needs/true self/soul as a poet with her willpower in the service of her ego or adaptive self—that is, being acceptable to others. The depressed person must be willing to depose the ego or will from its place of control because only the self has the embodied wisdom to take charge of the psyche. But, of course, the ego resists what is necessary because "the experience of the Self is always a defeat for the ego" (Jung, 1963, p. 546). Lewis spells out exactly how to listen to your true self and how to ignore your ego-driven will: "The only question to ask was 'is what I'm feeling real or fake?'" (2002, p. 169). We must find the strength to give time and space so that the listening soul "can hear the essence of things" (ibid., p. 126). As Lewis found: "Willpower is a good servant, but a bad master" (ibid., p. 128); it is not a renewable source of energy. (This echoes McGilchrist's (2010) contention that the big-picture, body-connected right brain should be the master, whereas the narrow-focus, abstracting left should be the emissary.) Likewise, in recovery, the will must be discarded: "Even though you'd do anything to make yourself feel better, part of the recovery is learning you can't" (Lewis, 2002, p. 204). How do you know what depression is telling you? Lewis is alive to its hints: what does it stop you doing? What does it force you to do in order to recover? What gives you more or less energy? When do you feel real? This is as much about *how* as what you are doing and being.

So, the depressed person must embrace his suffering and come to understand it as a defence against old wounds. What sort of things might depression be trying to tell the afflicted individual? Lessons about the past might involve mourning un-grieved losses, including early bereavements or neglectful, rejecting, or abusive parenting (e.g. Merkin, 2010; Slater, 1999). Many of the memoir writers remember happy childhoods in loving families, but may briefly mention parental depression such as maternal postnatal depression (e.g. Haig, 2015). By brushing this off as a one-liner, they show how little they understand the impact this would have had on them. Others remember a particular aspect of them being rejected, such as gender (Harding, 2013), sexual orientation (Solomon, 2014), or the drive towards autonomy and authenticity (McEvoy, 2011); such individuals must learn to fight the internalised parent for their right to be who they are. This may bring up a lot of anger and temporarily disturb the relationship to the (external) parent if he or she is still alive. Others still had such an unstable peripatetic childhood (Brampton,

2008) that they could never form secure attachments to friends, schools, homes, or even their families once they attained the age of going to boarding school. Such people need to work on forming stable, secure relationships and building a home, internally and externally. Some who have suffered early abuse have a very demanding task because the resulting trauma is probably hidden beneath a dissociation defence. Karla McLaren is a survivor of childhood sexual abuse, but in befriending her severe depression, she realised that: "The crippling lack of energy, focus, peace and happiness … wasn't the problem, and it didn't arise by mistake or accident; my energy was depleted because some part of me had sent it away on purpose—to keep it safe and alive until the end of my war" (2015, p. 29). Once again, depression is revealed to be not a pathology but an essential protection or survival strategy.

As we saw in Chapter 4, we learn to regulate emotions within the context of the early relationship with the mother. If, for any reason, she is inadequately attuned to our needs, we may instead come to suppress our affect or be emotionally overreactive. One of the primary tasks for such an individual in adult life is to learn affect regulation, which is accordingly a core purpose of psychotherapy (Schore, 2010). This was the case for Lorna Martin (2008), who managed her feelings through a mixture of suppressing or acting them out by means of competitive overwork, speeding, drink, and dysfunctional relationship. Her life was in a chaotic and obsessive downwards spiral with an underlying depression until she embarked on a year of thrice-weekly psychoanalytic psychotherapy. At the end, she was not only far more aware of her patterns, she was able to tolerate and withstand the strength of her feelings without acting out in response to them. Wurtzel (1996) and Jamison (1997) are notable among the memoirists in displaying even greater dysregulation than Martin, but neither of them report achieving a similar degree of regulation.

The depressed individual's current way of living is usually a defence or compensation for a fragile or fragmented self that was cobbled together in less than ideal conditions. For many of the memoir writers, the manic defence of non-stop work, socialising, and other activities ensured that they never had a crack in the flow of time through which self-awareness or self-reflection might creep in. But this is a very dangerous defence, in that it leads to chronic stress from excessive and conflicting commitments, all striving for the impossible: to guarantee safety, or to achieve perfection so as to bolster fragile self-esteem. In this manner we try to keep at bay the twin threats of abandonment and rejection. More generally, the insecurely attached defend against feeling because, as illustrated in the last paragraph, they have learned that feelings are dangerous and cannot be regulated. The nature of the infant/caregiver relationship generates the anxious attachment, fragile self, and sense of disconnection in the first place, and as we struggle to find ways to live from a crippled self, we replicate the old relationships. They are the ones that fit us, as the key fits the lock for which it was made. Depression may then herald a longing for authenticity, integration, or depth and a breaking free into safer, less dysregulating relationships where there is a capacity for both autonomy and intimacy.

The birth of the authentic self will entail letting go of some of the ego's compensating demands for fame, glory, or popularity, indeed most of what seems to be valued in our twenty-first-century culture. An episode of depression can be triggered when defences are punctured. For example, we may hold certain beliefs which we imagine will keep us safe and above criticism. We may believe that goodness will be rewarded, but undergo a shocking experience of the innocent being blamed or the guilty getting away with it. When such a constellated paradigm is invalidated, our entire world view is thrown into question (Rowe, 2003). Or we may find ourselves lapsing into depression after achieving a longed-for goal, like Richard Mabey (2006) when he completed his magnum opus *Flora Britannica*. This withdrawal can be caused by experiencing the emptiness of the self in the absence of the ego's goal, and/or by the achievement failing to bring the reward (love? admiration?) that was the unconscious motivation for the work in the first place. So an episode of depression or anxiety is a call to examine one's self, relationships and lifestyle, heal old wounds, and occupy untenanted spaces within ourselves.

Conclusion: conflict between needs versus goals, hopes, and expectations

Human beings have animal needs for survival and reproduction as well as specifically human needs—as described by Fromm (1990)—for relationship, creativity, rootedness, identity, and understanding. Depression arises from prolonged frustration of what Keedwell (2008) calls our archetypal needs. For most of the memoir writers the drive towards success was really a way of bolstering their identity, but there were a number of problems with their lifestyles that caused them to become depressed. First, they neglected their other needs, particularly for rest and leisure (health/survival needs), and, second, they fed only the ego part of their identities at the expense of a much deeper sense of authentic self. Keedwell shows how our goals can be incompatible with our needs for five different reasons: (1) incomplete understanding which makes it impossible to meet sets of needs that appear to conflict with each other; (2) moral inflexibility which either guarantees failure or leads to being ostracised from the peer group; (3) trying to please other people rather than yourself; (4) unrealistic goals and standards generated by overambitious parents or teachers; (5) a manic defence that covers up a sense of inner worthlessness. Most of the memoirists fit into the last three categories, all of which signal living out of the false self. Giving up on unrealistic goals—for which we don't have the interest, talent, or energy, or which conflict with other authentic needs—can in itself lead to the remission of depression (Keedwell, 2008). Sometimes, it is a matter of relinquishing the timing of events, like my client Ann who had a highly pressurising timetable for events in her life. Thus, each milestone immediately succeeded the next one so that there was never time for a rest, or to enjoy the last achievement: college, job, marriage, house, child, child, better house, third child, retirement to a smallholding by the age of forty. The purpose of depression is to force us to reassess how and why we continue to ignore, deny, and frustrate our needs. If we listen to its message, we can re-examine our drives and motivations and thereby realign ourselves with who we really are as distinct from what we are told is admirable by our society, or that to which our attachment patterns have habituated us.

In many cases the problem is not the individual, but it is society at large which is frustrating their needs. This was the case for several young clients who, in different ways, suffered from a void in meaning and values that meant they lacked any strong motivating goals in the first place (Dowds, 2018). In other cases, the social problems are material, so that the individual is trapped in a cycle of poverty, unemployment, or refugee status. They cannot permit themselves to have goals because they are aware of the overwhelming odds against succeeding in them. They are thus caught in a trap of helplessness and hopelessness.

CHAPTER 6

The therapeutic challenges of stuck mood

Which depressed patients benefit from psychotherapy

A large proportion of patients suffering major depression can link their symptoms to origins in psychosocial stress, but there are some exceptions. Some patients may have spent a lifetime free of this condition, but have a sudden onset of severe depression in later life. Some of these when followed up with a brain scan may be found to have had a stroke of which they are unaware. For example, damage to the left anterior prefrontal cortex is well known for inducing depression (Maletic & Raison, 2017). Physical problems such as chronic pain (with organic origins) or consumption of drugs or alcohol or withdrawal from them can all trigger depression (Dowds, 2018). For these latter patients, a primarily medical approach to treatment is called for, and psychotherapy is of limited value.

Not surprisingly, however, patients with a history of early-life adversity or dyadic discord (e.g. marriage problems) respond well to psychotherapy and less well to antidepressants (Maletic & Raison, 2017). Factors that contribute to client improvement in psychotherapy include client variables, the therapeutic relationship, model of therapy, and expectancy and placebo effects. Client factors are estimated to account for 40 per cent of improvement (average for all presenting issues), and successful treatment is associated with high motivation, a positive but realistic expectation of outcome and process, a readiness to change, and higher levels of psychological functioning (Cooper, 2008). In the case of therapy for depression, making a free choice for this type of treatment doubles the remission rate to fifty per cent (Maletic & Raison, 2017). Clients with personality disorders or insecure attachment, and who are perfectionist, are not psychologically minded or have low levels of social support, do less well in therapy overall (Cooper, 2008). Unfortunately, this collection of adverse attributes is virtually a checklist for the psychodynamics of the depressed client. Clients who ruminate show a poorer response to CBT but benefit from mindfulness-based approaches: attention is refocused from the past to the present, and questions and judgements give way to acceptance (Maletic & Raison, 2017).

Psychotherapy—unlike antidepressants—is long-lasting and prevents relapse. It severs the abnormal connection of the executive network to the default mode network and strengthens its connection to the salience network (ibid.). However, it must be remembered that depression is not just low mood but also *stuck mood*. Traumatised clients—many of whom succumb to depression—are prone to hyperarousal by activation of the SNS, or hypo-arousal via the dorsal vagus, or they oscillate between the two, and they tend to have a narrow window of tolerance for processing emotional input (Ogden et al., 2006). For this reason, depressed clients are often rigid and resistant to therapeutic engagement. The stuckness and rigidity must be slowly and gently challenged before the client can engage in depth psychotherapy. This chapter focuses on working with these blocks.

Which therapies are best for depression?

The conventional view is that CBT, sometimes coupled with mindfulness meditation, is the therapy of choice for depression. A great deal more research has been done on CBT than on other approaches, and CBT has indeed been found to be at least as effective as antidepressants, with lower relapse rates (Cooper, 2008). However, absence of evidence should not be confused with absence of effect, and when CBT has been compared with other psychotherapies, they have usually been found to have similar efficacy in the treatment of depression. When CBT was compared with non-directive therapy, the reduction in BDI (Beck Depression Inventory) scores was virtually identical in the space of four months (ibid.). Likewise, interpersonal therapy and CBT were found to be equally effective over sixteen sessions (ibid.). This suggests that it is common factors such as the therapeutic relationship that have the biggest impact on the client, and indeed it has been demonstrated that technique/therapy model effects account for only 15 per cent of improvement in psychotherapy in general (Asay & Lambert, 1999). However, while virtually all comparative studies show equivalence in outcome between different therapeutic approaches, these are average results. They do not imply that all therapies are equal for individual clients or specific client groups. In the case of phobias and panic disorders, for example, the CBT technique of in vivo exposure has been shown to be particularly useful (Cooper, 2008). Furthermore, different approaches may have different long-term outcomes, and one recent study has shown that the gains of psychoanalytic psychotherapy lasted for at least two years post-treatment, whereas the benefits of CBT failed to be maintained (Fonagy et al., 2015).

One neuroscientifically informed model of depression conceives of it as an attractor state caused by not receiving expected rewards, or by receiving punishers (Rolls, 2018). This researcher proposes behavioural treatments such as engaging in tasks that require a lot of attention (e.g. sailing or golf)—thereby inhibiting rumination—or activities that lead to reward. Before deciding on appropriate tasks, it is of course necessary to know the type of non-reward or punisher that led to the depression in the first place. If it was the death of a much-loved partner, continued focus on the loss may bring on depression, whereas a celebration of the life of the deceased or taking account of all they brought to the life of the bereaved one may compete with the "non-reward attractor". Ultimately it may be possible to move on to new relationships or a new way of living that bring rewards that the previous relationship did not.

Problems specific to working with depression

It might be assumed from the preceding chapters that working with depression is straightforward: one needs to work on the trauma or the insecure attachment and build a flexible and embodied sense of self that is secure in relationship. To be sure, none of these building blocks come easily, but they are the stuff of normal psychodynamically informed psychotherapy. So why is depression in a special category of its own?

Depression is a learned response to a given situation, but as time passes it becomes, like any engrained pattern, habitual. It becomes inbuilt into neural pathways and mental states: the repeated activation of a state of sadness, shame, or despair (for example) makes them easier to activate in the future, like a path being trodden through grass, and when such *states* of mind become habitual, they become *traits* of the individual. Using complexity theory, Daniel Siegel has argued that organisation of the self requires both differentiation and linkage of its elements. Healthy (i.e. complex) self-organisation results in a flexible self, capable of responding appropriately to current conditions in the environment, where complexity depends on "a balance between the continuity and the flexibility of the system" (Siegel, 2012, p. 197). On the other hand, poor organisation results in either rigidity (too much continuity, e.g. depression) or chaos (too much flexibility, e.g. mania). It is this rigidity in depressed clients that makes them so difficult to work with: it manifests in cognitive, emotional, and energetic fixity that resists the therapist's efforts to promote change, because these are experienced as a threat to the continuity of the self.

A complex system needs, as Siegel argues, both differentiation of parts and linkage between them. People who are insecurely attached either lack differentiation in relationship to others (too closely matched in communication: ambivalent types) or they lack linkage (unmatched in communication: avoidant types) or both (disorganised attachment) and thus have relatively non-integrated mental states which remain stuck in past ways of being and respond inappropriately to the present situation (Beebe et al., 2005). Securely attached pairs display a balance between matching the other and having the freedom to vary responses. It is striking that the parents of avoidantly attached children have poor affect attunement and communicate with little facial expression: this is what the avoidant child learns. In states of depression there is a loss of this capacity for processing facial affect (Siegel, 2012).

Another way of understanding the fixed state is to see it as one of the responses to threat: not fight or flight, but freeze. This corresponds to a theory of the evolutionary origins of depressive behaviour as a defence for young animals whose mothers have left them to go hunting or grazing, or who have been killed. The isolated baby has the best chance of survival if it stays very still, thus conserving its energy resources and not drawing the attention of predators. Freezing is in general the last-ditch response to threat where neither fight nor flight are feasible: a young child can neither challenge nor leave an overwhelming parent.

Complex systems are non-linear, so that "a small change in input can lead to huge and unpredictable changes in outcome" (Siegel, 2012, p. 199). This means in principle that in therapy it may be possible to have an enormous change from a tiny intervention, as I myself have occasionally experienced. In the most extreme example, a woman client spoke of how she was torturing herself with guilt, anxiety, and excessive responsibility in relationship to others in her wide circle of family, friends, and neighbours. When I asked her to tune into what she was experiencing in the front of her body, she was shocked to feel the knot in her stomach and to realise that it was always there. Once she got in touch with this, she was sufficiently appalled to simply stop this over-focus on others at the expense of herself. Her life became transformed in an apparently stable manner. However, I have had the opposite experience with depressed clients who are so buried in past ways of being and relating that it is very difficult to "figure out which system changes are needed in order to alter the constraints on rigidly engrained attractor states" (Siegel, 2012, p. 200). Most of our contact with others occurs unconsciously, and Allan Schore (2010) has argued that it is in this implicit engagement between the right hemispheres of the client and therapist that transformative therapy takes place. This implies that our countertransferential responses are of most significance in therapy: what we are picking up in our bodies about the client facing us.

Anyone who has worked with depressed clients knows that many of them actively block the therapist's attempts to induce change. Why do they do this? Many have a belief that change is not possible: a belief that is remarkably resistant to rational argument. The fixed beliefs (see Table 6.1) that are characteristic of depressed clients are probably a defence against something even worse than depression. What might be worse? One is the anxiety that is the flip side of the depression coin. If nothing matters on the depression side so that life isn't worth living,

Table 6.1

Rigid beliefs in depressed clients

This is the way I am, i.e. nothing will ever change

This is the way other people are … and there is only one possible response to them

Individuals are either good or bad, right or wrong (splitting)

Disturbances in relationships are exclusively caused by my shortcomings

Disturbances in relationships are exclusively caused by the other's shortcomings

Rifts in relationships can't be healed so all I can do is walk away

There is only one way to interpret events (intolerance of ambiguity)

I should be able to achieve anything if I work hard enough/I'm useless (unrealistic appraisal of chance of reaching goals)

I am responsible even for events beyond my control

It is my duty to protect others and I have no right to take care of myself

I must feel/think/do what my family/friends/colleagues want (inhibition of independent thinking)

then on the anxiety side, everything matters too much so that life can't be lived (Dowds, 2018). One client flipped back and forth between dismissing all her relationships as worthless and them mattering so much that she couldn't leave the house for fear of the humiliating things her acquaintances might see and gossip about: "I saw Nicky today. Still no job, still hanging round with those losers, you know the ones who hang round the town centre smoking dope." In such a case of depression linked to social anxiety there is no sense of relationship as an ongoing process, no model of the repair of ruptures in attunement. These clients cannot question, explore, or check out whether a comment they have taken as shaming was indeed intended as such. Experiencing insult means insult was intended: the only possible response is schism and cut-off in the relationship.

The rigid beliefs of clients about their lives inevitably follow them into the therapy room in a series of self-frustrating patterns (Table 6.2). For example, many depressed clients are terrified of hope awakening, followed by the inevitable (as they see it) devastation as their hopes

Table 6.2

Self-frustrating patterns in depression

Inhibition of feelings: anger, assertiveness, aliveness, curiosity, sexual interest, etc.

Investment in feeling worthless—protecting the attachment relationship at the expense of my own self-esteem

Investment in guilt—I would be a bad/selfish person if I didn't feel guilty

Not letting go—problem with partial grieving because to let go would be a betrayal

Investment in being helpless or ill because these were the only times I was ever cared for

Self-isolating because relationships are associated with terror, rage, anxiety, shaming, etc.

Perfectionism—this is the only way I can be respected

---

are dashed. They prefer to remain depressed than to face such crushing disappointment. For others the pain of their worthlessness or shame is so excruciating the wound cannot be touched. They are incapable of working close up to such agony—there is no window of tolerance—and prefer to hang on to their state of numbness. In some cases the pain is physical, as recounted in some depression memoirs—the burning sensation experienced by Wolpert (1999); agony "worse than tearing in childbirth with a faulty epidural" (Kelly, 2014, p. 25)—which makes attention to therapy virtually impossible.

Many depressed clients are invested in holding on to their shame, guilt, helplessness, isolation, or perfectionism because their beliefs or experience tell them that something worse will be felt if they let go. Attacking these beliefs will only create a split between the left brain and the embodied emotions. Rather it is essential to explore the fears that underlie each belief.

Therapy with depressed clients

When working with depressed clients, it is crucial to be aware that depression is a defence against something worse: anxiety, terror, unbearable pain (e.g. from rejection or shame), or sometimes unmanageable rage.

Therefore, it is understandable that attempts to strip the client of the depression too quickly will be met with resistance. Thus the therapist can feel in a double-bind: the client is desperate for your help but won't (can't) accept anything you have to offer—they just want immediate relief of symptoms. There is of course a place for antidepressant medication here, and for some CBT exercises: these include breaking down global statements into specifics; challenging various kinds of negative thinking, including catastrophising; learning to tolerate ambiguity; countering behavioural patterns; becoming aware of the triggers for negative feelings (see Leahy et al., 2011; Wills, 2008). But the problem with CBT is that it is resolutely anchored in the present moment and in the conscious mind and conceives of clients as broken machines within which rational cognition needs to be reasserted. As such it lacks the psychic depth, emotional awareness, inspiration, imagination, embodiment, and focus on relationship that depressed clients desperately need. Depending on the client's world view, they may find CBT either reassuring, or deeply limited and even offensively mechanical.

Before exploring ways of disrupting low motivation in therapy, let us establish what our aim is in the treatment of depression. I am reminded of the statement of Steve Porges that, for trauma, "safety is the treatment" (Badenoch, 2018, p. 78). This means providing the client with the essential relational conditions for surviving and thriving: conditions that are available to them perhaps for the first time in their lives. What this might be for the depressed client depends on what childhood adversities made them vulnerable to depression in the first place. Thus, the client may need not to be exposed, put on the spot, asked to do what they can't—therefore creative approaches need to be negotiated sensitively. In general, the therapist must be alive to how the effects of early abuse or neglect manifests for the client in the present. A lot of attention must go into attuned listening, sensitive responsiveness, and repair of ruptures in relatedness. In drawing attention to the dangers of being led by techniques, I can't do better than to quote Bonnie Badenoch:

> If I open the door to greet my patient with my own idea about which technique will best help this person, my ventral vagal parasympathetic will most likely be offline, a condition that will

communicate lack of safety to my client. Probably none of this will rise to a level of conscious awareness, but it will cause a neu-roception of lack of connection and therefore danger, influencing what will unfold between us. (2018, p. 81)

It is absolutely vital to foreground the relationship, so that any tech-niques (e.g. working with parts) that are used arise spontaneously out of the present moment in the client's process.

Developing detachment

Depressed people are often overwhelmed by painful feelings and can only work on the experience when a little detachment is developed between the aware self and the thoughts and feelings of depression. The depression can be externalised in various ways, such as viewing it on a cinema screen with the client in the audience watching it. Alternatively, in Siegel's wheel of awareness (2010), the client can visualise his or her aware consciousness at the hub of a wheel, while on different sectors of the rim are external physical sensations, internal (proprioceptive) sensa-tions, feelings, thoughts, memories, fantasies, beliefs, etc. The depressed client who observes her despair on the rim of the wheel gets a feeling of spaciousness and can tolerate it since she is no longer drowning in it. There are many other projective techniques such as drawing; work-ing with dolls/puppets; or exploring the client's reactions to paintings of depressed subjects, depressing themes, or even abstract forms. When working with paintings or other images, the therapist encourages the client to tell the story of what they project onto the image, and then they play with possible conclusions or endings.

Disrupting low motivation

The best way I know of getting beyond the frozen rigidity of depres-sion is to separate out the parts (subpersonalities) that are fused together: e.g. the part that believes nothing will ever change versus a small nub of hope that has brought the client into therapy (Fisher, 2017; Mearns & Thorne, 2000; Rowan, 1990; Schwartz, 2001). This can be done using a combination of voice dialogue, body therapy, and a variety of creative techniques: dolls, art work, dramatisation of the parts, visualisation techniques, as well as mindfulness practice that distances the parts away from the centre of consciousness (see above).

For clients who believe that when they try, they will fail or otherwise get hurt, the initial need is to disrupt their low motivation before they will commit to therapy. How can we transform low motivation? The internal family systems work developed by Richard Schwartz (2001) enables the client to understand the multiple, dissonant parts of the self and, crucially, to disidentify from the parts. As long as we identify with the part, curiosity and interest about it are impossible (Fisher, 2017). One way of working is to find the body locus of the low motivation and enter into a dialogue with it. Generally, it plays a numbing role to protect exiled parts that are hurt. These parts may carry pain, shame, or terror, and the client naturally resists opening them up and feeling the acute pain under the numbing defence. The therapist must ask permission of the protector part of the client to work with the exiled parts. Find out how the client feels about the hurt part until they move beyond hatred or shame about it, towards also finding curiosity, compassion, courage, or any other positive emotion that will help them to engage with the part. Then ask the client about the past and how the part was hurt and abandoned. Finally ask the adult self to help the inner child. It can be useful to use dolls or puppets to help the parts come alive.

It is crucial in this work to welcome *all* of the parts of the client (including the hopeless part) and to allow the apparently unhelpful and initially dominant negative voices to exhaust what they have to say. Then, when a small cue appears ("but I did have a moment of lightness on Sunday morning when I saw the daffodil shoots appearing—they seemed like a moment of hope"), gently move into curiosity about this part. It is usually a revelation and liberation for the client when they experience the difference between "I am depressed" and "this part of me has withdrawn because it was so hurt in the past".

Two of the positive basic emotions of PLAY and SEEKING (Panksepp, 2010) are particularly diminished in depressed people. Representing parts with toys, art work, or dramatic enactments maps a route into the joy of play, which in itself has antidepressant effects. A way of engaging the seeking impulse is described in the following section.

Opening up perspective

Depressed clients tend, as we have seen, to have a very narrow and fixed focus and to feel stuck in an unchangeable present. One way of opening them up is by visualisation: get them to imagine their depressed mind state as an island or a park bench, then encourage them to spread their attention to the wider world beyond the island, or to the rest of the park beyond the bench. Working metaphorically, the client can describe what they see: trees, lake, ducks, buildings, cinemas, cafes, other people, and so on. How do they feel when they take on this broader perspective? What does this mean for their own lives? This is where the reasons for the depression may enter the dialogue in terms of difficult relationships, which evoke humiliation, shame, guilt, fear, etc. But in that wider world, they may also be able to find sources of joy or meaning.

In depression, the basic emotion of SEEKING (Panksepp, 2010) has become muted or crushed. This is the emotion associated with exploration, libido, and learning, with all the intense engagement with life that has been withdrawn in the depressed person. It is possible to reawaken it through visualisation, for example, exploring back alleyways and junk shops in an old city. There are some creative ideas for exploring, experimenting and experiencing in Stevens (1989); better still, tailor-make visualisations for the specific client which helps them connect with their strengths and enriches them with what they are lacking, while at the same time gently helping them to engage with the source of their pain.

Starting to breathe deeply

The depressed client is generally torpid in movement and restricted in their breathing and, as we noted above, they have lost the capacity for playing or never developed it in the first place. Exercise has been shown to be very beneficial to enliven the client and can be initiated within the therapy room. Depending on the dyad and the space available, stretching and various bioenergetic movements can be done (e.g. trudging like a depressed person followed by light-hearted skipping along), or dancing or singing could form part of the therapy, or games such as pushing, cushion fights, or mock sword-fights can be created for clients out of touch with their aggression, playfulness, or boundaries. The therapist can also help the client design an exercise regime outside the therapy room that will suit his physical and emotional capacities and needs. For the isolated client, group exercise is useful and for one who is artistic rather than sporty, dancing classes or singing in a choir may be the answer. Martial arts build confidence, yoga holds a space for relaxation, while pilates centres and strengthens. Engaging the client in creating movement or in breathing exercises empowers them as they become more aware of and able to assert both their physiological demands and their psychosocial needs vis-à-vis other people. As a caveat, the nature and origins of the blocks to deep breathing need to be respected and explored. Indeed, a sudden deepening of breath could generate anxiety, even a panic attack.

Completing the unmetabolised experience

Stuck moods like depression and anxiety overlay repeated unmetabolised experiences (Ogden et al., 2006). Thus yearning, or rage, or assertion of boundaries may have been blocked in early life. As the client remembers incidents from childhood and begins to go into a shutdown state, the therapist can gently intervene, slow down the withdrawal, and invite the client to be open to another pathway. If the client's depression is a long-term freeze state (in response to childhood threat), they may move into fight or flight; if it is a longing for intimacy as in insecure attachment, they may move towards opening their arms and their hearts. The work here should focus on the body and what *it* wants to do *now*: feel the emotion and tension and act it out symbolically (e.g. walk out of the door, or strangle, thump, kick, or hug a cushion). The main thing for the therapist is to catch and slow down that liminal moment where the path hitherto not taken may be tested.

Uncovering depression's purpose

Learning from depression has been explored in Chapter 5; this section is simply a reminder of how the therapist can guide this process. The crucial questions are: "What message does the depression contain?", "What does it want?", "What is its purpose?", or whatever formulation works for the particular client. When the depression is projected onto a cinema screen or through the use of any of the creative approaches already mentioned, the answers to the central question may emerge. By exploring the figures or symbols on the screen, the client's psychosocial issues become clearer: treating himself like a thing without rest or mercy; engaging in relationships which deplete the sense of self; believing that she is a failure; feeling alienated or threatened in a toxic corporate environment; living with a heart frozen from lack of intimacy, or broken from loss of the natural world—and many other variants of fundamental human needs that are not being met (Dowds, 2018). The current triggers can then be traced back to various kinds of stress or grief in childhood including insecure attachment.

Disrupting the internal focus

Many clients who have little self-awareness need to be encouraged to develop it as in traditional psychotherapy. However, there are others who are already far too preoccupied with their inner process and need to start looking outside themselves. This can be done in an infinity of ways: for example, through helping others, playing like or with a child or animal, exploring a topic or a landscape, travelling, camping in nature, gardening, music, or externally focused meditation.

For people who analyse (with the left hemisphere) their feelings endlessly but fruitlessly (rumination), it may be helpful for them to engage with their feelings in a more creative way, such as through art work, movement, making up a story. They would also benefit from the reframing offered by psychosynthesis: converting the mantra of "I am depressed" into "I am sometimes visited by depression, but my sadness or shame are not who I am". Another powerful way to release obsessive thoughts is through mindfulness meditation practice (Pedulla, 2016; Roemer & Orsillo, 2016).

Working with relationships

While building a trusting relationship in the therapy room is all-important, if shame is a huge issue, it will be necessary to set up the room so that eye contact is not forced on the client. However, at some stage this must be challenged, perhaps through play; otherwise the blocks to contact will never be healed. Having a shared focus for the dyad such as paintings or client photographs, or even a pet—belonging to the therapist or the client—can be helpful intermediaries, where contact can be made through a third non-threatening object. Likewise, in the outside world, acquiring a dog may help the isolated client form his first trusting relationship, provide exercise through walking the dog, and the beginnings of human contact through talking to other dog walkers.

For the client living with a partner, the relationship can sometimes contribute to generating or maintaining depression. Dorothy Rowe has shown various ways in which the identified patient is simply playing their part in the family system. For example, "sometimes what the 'well' partner needs is to be needed, and the 'ill' partner obligingly meets this need" (Rowe, 2003, p. 187). Such depressogenic relational patterns can include the partner being abusive, neglectful, controlling, manipulative, or colluding with the depressed person's withdrawal, compliance, hyper-independence etc. In such cases, couple therapy is indicated.

Conclusion

The apparent resistance of depressed clients to therapy is in reality both a necessary defence and a pointer to their underlying wound. Therefore, the early stages of therapy must focus on building a relationship and fostering some trust and hope in the client. Their fixed belief that they have an unchangeable affliction can be questioned once they have small sensations of aliveness, perhaps as they begin to complete old unmetabolised experiences. This can help them to understand the message held in their depression. What worse thing is being defended against? What is the depression asking of the client in relation to their current way of being in the world? How can they move out of themselves and learn to build safe and satisfying relationships?

CHAPTER 7

Repairing the self, building resilience

One reason why depression is so complex to work with is that it is experienced at multiple levels simultaneously: through the body, the emotions, thoughts, and existential world view/meaning, as well as in relationship. The therapist must engage all levels, often at the same time, while maintaining awareness that it was usually the nature of early relationships, particularly the primary attachments, that generated the patterns in the first place. For the sake of presentation, these factors are separated out in the following sections; but in the consulting room, all elements must be given their place. At any one moment, one or other of the elements may be foregrounded: some sessions may be primarily somatic, others psychodynamic, some may focus on present-day anxiety, some on attachment patterns, others on beliefs. This chapter will emphasise client issues rather than techniques. It is useless to concoct a toolkit of ready-made techniques because any intervention that is attuned to the moment will emerge spontaneously within the session. Interventions must always be a response to clients (though sometimes to an absence in them), never a pre-emptive impingement. With some clients, I occasionally use projective/creative methods, meditative approaches, or body/voice work; with others I "just" listen and respond.

Research has shown that "security priming" improves subjects' moods, even in the face of a threat. These methods include subliminal messages with the names of people who enhance security, or images suggesting that an attachment figure is available to them, and—more usefully for the practitioner—guided imagery about how available and supportive such safe attachment figures are (Mikulincer & Shaver, 2013). Clients who experienced their therapists as sensitive and supportive were more likely to get relief from depression and to maintain the benefits of therapy over an eighteen-month period (Zuroff & Blatt, 2006).

Working with insecure attachment

When a client presents with depression, it can be useful to focus on issues of negative models of self; negative models of other; and patterns of emotional and somatic (mal)adaptation to the environment, including affect regulation and emotional defences. The content and process of therapy will be influenced by the client's self-loathing; their mistrust, fear, or dependence on the other; their denial, suppression of or other defences against feeling; or their being highly reactive or numbed out in regulating affect. The therapist and client must agree on issues and goals, create a relatively safe, secure, and stable alliance, and begin to track patterns of emotional processing and interpersonal engagement. A combination of feedback and questioning helps to make emotions more explicit and specific, while the felt sense (through Gendlin's body focusing) helps the client to experience them in an embodied way (Gendlin, 1996). This is important for ruminating clients "stuck in their heads", who can easily gain in self-awareness at an intellectual level without anything ever changing. With such individuals, interpretation and understanding may often serve to strengthen the intellectual defence and remove them even further from *embodied experiencing* of their feelings. At the end of this initial stage of therapy, the client should be more regulated emotionally (less reactive or numbed out), more discovery oriented about their inner experience, able to recognise their relational patterns, and more able to integrate their responses into a meaningful narrative (Johnson, 2019).

At the next stage of attachment therapy, the task for the therapist is to gently challenge the client (e.g. through repetition and images) to face experiences of longing, abandonment, rejection, isolation, and emptiness: possibly starting with key adult relationships, but then moving back into childhood. These may be accompanied by intense, even cata-strophic emotions, particularly panic, sadness, and shame. The therapist needs to provide a safe and secure presence, with consistent holding, pro-tection against emotional overwhelm, mirroring of feelings and accurate psycho-feedback, all of which were compromised in the original attach-ment relationship: "*Vulnerability is embraced and owned in a way that leaves the client feeling more whole and more balanced, and ironically, more powerful*" (Johnson, 2019, p. 91, italics in original). Ultimately, new patterns of response can emerge in terms of the client's model of self, other, and relationship. For example, to the degree that the ambivalently attached individual consciously faces the terror of abandonment, they become less dependent on the other; when the avoidant can face the rage and shame at being consistently misunderstood, at their feelings being disparaged or ignored, and their dependency treated with contempt or irritation, they are able to develop more tolerance for closeness. As inner emptiness is confronted, a new emotional resilience can permit the self to develop and relate more securely to adult attachment figures. (See Johnson, 2019 for detailed dialogues representing stages in the attach-ment therapy process.)

The relationship between therapist and client will inevitably throw up parallels to the childhood attachment relationship. This may be viewed, not so much in terms of transference, but as a real-life and present-time re-enactment of attachment patterns. The points at which contact between the dyad are broken highlight the key relational issues. The therapist should be capable of sensitive attunement and mentaliza-tion, but problems are bound to arise, such as misunderstanding, and perceived abandonment and rejection. It is crucial that the therapist be willing and able to repair ruptures in attunement, while accepting that mistakes are inevitable and not a cause for guilt. The therapist must be able to model what is most difficult for the client: being present and in contact with the other while retaining a sense of self; tolerating stress and uncertainty; and having a capacity for self-care.

Loss and grief

I am so far in that I can see no end/ and no distance: everything has become close/ and everything close has turned to stone. R. M. Rilke, from *Das Stundenbuch* (translated by Peter Labanyi).

In this poem about grief, Rilke evokes its similarity to depression in all its stuckness and ruminating narrowness. Bereavement is frequently followed by depression, particularly when social support is lacking. Indeed, it has been argued that there is little difference between depression and loss-related grief, except that the latter is more expected and socially accepted (Dowds, 2018).

When the presenting issue is loss of an attachment partner, therapy may evolve from support in the grieving process to engaging with questions about identity, self, and relationships. The bereaved person has literally lost a part of their world: they experience the loneliness of having nobody there to share their lives, from trivial events to a holiday or a major life experience. Indeed, the person they most need to get them through the bereavement may be the very person they have lost. Widowed and divorced/separated people frequently suffer further losses, such as friends whose loyalty lies with the dead or separated spouse. Loss may be followed by a normal and healthy period of grieving, at the end of which we make the loss a part of our lives. However, sometimes mourning is unresolved and turns into melancholia—depression—as Freud described in his classic "Mourning and Melancholia" (1917e). It may be impossible to complete the process of grieving because of guilt about old hurts, hatreds, or resentments towards the dead person. It is too late for reparation and so the individual cannot move on. This is similar to the stasis which besets some people in their own dying when they have uncompleted business with the living: they cannot let go into death until the unspoken has been acknowledged (Kearney, 1996).

What does mourning need to accomplish, asks the Lacanian Darian Leader (2009)? He suggests that four tasks must be completed to arrive at acceptance of loss. The first is the creation of a symbolic space of transition which is often revealed in dreams, in the form of doorways, arches, or stages, etc. The second involves the symbolic killing of the dead person, whether consciously through ritual in traditional cultures, or unconsciously in dreams for the modern mourner. The wake is a mourning ritual which is still extant in rural Ireland. By having a party around the open coffin, the wake celebrates the life of the deceased while also integrating the bereaved family members back into the community in their new identity. The folk tradition is replete with songs and stories about the corpse awakening in the coffin, keeping alive the hope, or fear, that the deceased is not dead after all, and may need to be returned to their own realm.

Sometimes it is impossible for us to let the loved one go because of a sense of loyalty to them. We may believe that we are indebted to the dead for what they gave us, or for what we failed to give them. One father whose grief for his son was as raw ten years later as at the time of death refused to seek help in the form of therapy. He feared perhaps the deconstruction of his idealised picture of their relationship, and possibly facing the guilt at how his wild, uncontained parenting had played its part in his son's death in a motorcycle accident. He needs to face the fact that some debts are unpayable.

The third element of mourning concerns separating out the person we have lost from what we have lost in them—to use the terminology of self-psychology, the self-object they were for us. This is made particularly difficult when the mourner's love is of a narcissistic kind—grieving for someone who reflected who I am or how I would like to be seen, maybe as the wife of a man of status. Then letting go of them is letting go of ourselves, and we must "sacrifice … our own links to the image" (ibid., p. 135). This sacrifice may be symbolised, perhaps by a lock of the mourner's hair thrown into the grave with the dead.

The fourth strand of the mourning process requires us to mourn who we were for the dead person. Who else will ever love me as my dead husband did? Who else will privilege me as my mother did? As Joan Didion poignantly noted following the death of her husband: "For forty years I saw myself through John's eyes. … This year for the first time since I was twenty-nine I saw myself through the eyes of others" (2006, p. 197). In a loving marriage, the eyes of the spouse are much more forgiving than the eyes of the world—and it is hard to imagine how we can survive in this harsh and cruel new environment. When grief turns into depression, the individual may withdraw from this non-adapting and unsympathetic world (rather like Japanese *hikikomori* who retreat to their bedrooms).

Anxiety

One way of understanding depression is as a defence against anxiety, often brought on by excessive stress (Dowds, 2018; Rowe, 2003). For this reason, anxiety is often the primary mood presented by the depressed client. The discussion below refers to non-traumatised clients. In cases of trauma, the causes of anxiety are more profound and challenging.

I generally find that there are commonly four interrelated issues that need to be tackled simultaneously to soothe anxiety. First, the client's pace of life must slow down. This is easily stated, but is usually met with resistance by clients because their source of meaning and their defence against an empty sense of self is intimately tied up with achievements, future plans, and/or entangled relationships. Interconnected with the first goal is a second of living more in the present and less in the future. Naturally, exhortations to live in the present moment are met with a deaf ear because what this entails for the individual is not only experiencing the anxiety itself, but also uncovering her inner emptiness. The third task is to get in touch with their somatic responses to situations along with bodily impulses that are associated with the positive and negative emotions. This goal of embodiment is the most important of the three and underpins the success of the others. Some people are so disconnected from their bodies that they cannot even see the point of embodiment. However, they find, as they gradually become aware of their stomach or their breathing responses to stressful situations (for example), they can no longer override their body messages as they did before. All of this work will be met with a barrage of "yes, buts" which must be countered with patient acceptance until there is spontaneous movement. There are no quick fixes, and all of the above require constant practice, a moment-by-moment mindfulness of how they are living. It is important to emphasise that these changes cannot be made by attending therapy for an hour a week, or even by a daily mindfulness meditation. They must be incorporated into all the complexity and pressure of a lived life, not sequestered off into some daily or weekly quality time with oneself. At the same time, this moment-by-moment process of somatic experiencing needs therapy to provide support, the development of awareness, and learning within a reparative relationship. The speediness, future-orientation, and disembodiment being challenged here are all defences against a weak sense of self that have started to work against the client. Thus, strengthening the self is the ultimate goal of therapy.

Chronic fear in relationships—of rejection, judgement, or impingement—is the fourth component of many people's anxiety.

This drives such clients towards people-pleasing or distancing in relationships, but these coping strategies inevitably generate their own stresses and anxieties. Depending on their type of insecure attachment, some people feel weak and emotionally dependent, while others believe that there is nobody they can trust. Both patterns generate abandonment anxiety, the former fearing imminent abandonment, the latter having accepted in infancy that they are alone in regulating their emotions and meeting their other needs. The former ambivalent types have weak boundaries against others and feel controlled by their perceived needs, wishes, or demands. The latter avoidant types have rigid boundaries and may feel primarily depressed rather than anxious, because of their loneliness, isolation, and fear of intimacy. Attachment anxiety may be triggered by loss (e.g. of job or relationship), or by stress caused by the defence itself. Both types can be worked with by expanding the client's window of tolerance for closeness (avoidant) or separateness (ambivalent). Through achieving more healthy ways of relating (gaining capacities for autonomy and intimacy), the client works indirectly on his weak sense of self.

Therapy for fragile, false, or fragmented self

Depression is often underpinned by having a poorly developed sense of self, inadequate relationships with parents in childhood and therefore with subsequent attachment figures in later life, as well as by a sense of existential meaninglessness (Dowds, 2018). In reality these are all linked: the fragile self is a consequence of and later sustained by poor relationships, and meaninglessness a consequence of the deficits of self: "The search for meaning … is actually the search for the essence of the self" (Almaas, 2001, p. 228). The weak sense of self lays the foundations for greater sensitivity to stress, anxiety, and depression as well as difficulties with later relationships, while social conditions of isolation, stress, and loss in the modern urban and globalised world exacerbate early childhood vulnerabilities.

Depth psychotherapy involves developing the fragile self and a new way of relating to others as well as becoming aware of current unsustainable and unnourishing ways of living. Depressed individuals must learn to relate with both boundaries and a capacity for intimacy, and they must develop awareness of their authentic organismic impulses as a precursor to forming a stronger more integrated sense of self. In working with clients in touch with early childhood, it is crucial to remember that their experiences at the time were emotional, somatic, and preverbal, which is why therapy should target the right hemisphere of the client (Schore, 2010). Healing of such early material requires relating to the child and adult parts of the individual simultaneously. As one therapist put it: "I keep in mind that I am talking to patients not so much verbally as preverbally. I use the verbal communication as a means of carrying inflection and an accompaniment of facial expression and postural components" (quoted in Coyne, 1985, p. 326).

No amount of CBT will give you the self that is missing: it simply addresses the elimination of symptoms. Nor can meditation, even when practised over a long period of time, replace depth psychotherapy. According to Cortright, meditation and therapy do two quite different things, neither of which substitutes for the other, though they can enhance each other (Dowds, 2018). He concludes that while most types of meditation do promote relaxation, for the majority of people their "defences and neuroses are relatively intact after sustained meditation practice" (1997, p. 151).

Therapy for depression must be exploratory—of the client's unconscious as well as their conscious adaptations. While this can be achieved in psychoanalytic and humanistic and integrative therapies, the former may be suitable only for those who start with a lot of interiority and have less need of reparative relationship. The more engaged relational style in humanistic therapies may be more appropriate for those who have attunement and mirroring deficits. A warning note against traditional psychoanalysis is sounded by Verhaeghe (2008), who has observed a new kind of patient in his practice. Most of these suffer from anxiety and depression but with no obvious immediate cause, "where the most insignificant drawback is enough to trigger the depression [and anxiety] that [are] already there" (p. 5). Since there is nothing to dismantle in these patients, psychoanalytic approaches must move beyond deconstruction to actively and experientially working with—not just talking about—the dynamics of relating.

In the case of the narcissistic kind of fragile self, Almaas says the wound must be both experienced and understood to grasp its relationship to inadequate mirroring and "losing sight of what is genuine in us" (2001, p. 317). For failures in the development of self organisation, therapy must also be reparative, to substitute for the parental relationship that was less than good enough. It has been clear for some decades now that the self develops only in relationships, and that its qualities of strength, stability, resilience, and flexibility are dependent on the quality of the primary relationship. Classical psychoanalysis of the kind that frustrates the client by refusing to meet their developmental needs undermines precisely this requirement for relationship. In developing self-psychology, Kohut was motivated by his awareness that patients with a weak sense of self needed empathy rather than interpretation from the analyst. Cooper, writing of Kohut's views on therapy concludes: "The objective inspectional, inferential stance of the analyst contributes to a consistent attitude of muted responsiveness, which for many narcissistic characters in analysis imposes a repetition of the deprivation circumstance—that is, the lack of empathy for the patient's need for vividness, responsiveness, and so forth, which were the original source of the developmental failure" (1986, p. 135).

This applies equally to any kind of failure in self formation, whether empty, fragmented, or false self (Dowds, 2018). In Kohut's terms, the therapist must allow the mirror and/or idealising transferences: he or she must "consistently maintain the empathic rather than objective stance" (Cooper, 1986, p. 136). In person-centred terms, the therapist's task is to provide Rogers' (1967) core conditions of empathy, congruence, and positive regard. A more integrative updating of optimum therapy conditions—informed by infant observation research—applies the *intersubjective* nature of mother-child communication to the therapist–client relationship (Mearns & Cooper, 2005; Nolan, 2012; Pearmain, 2001).

Frosh pinpoints the relational process whereby psychoanalytic psychotherapy heals the conflicted, fragmented self, a description that could equally apply to humanistic and integrative therapy:

> Taking in, holding, making sense, giving back—this is the process of containment, resulting from the state of reverie. From the point of view of the infant or patient, the experience of such a containment is of having one's fragmented self, with all its destructive elements, accepted, tolerated and made manageable, alongside an awareness that this beneficial cycle arises from the presence of a holding, reliable and patient other. (1991, p. 185)

To use Toni Morrison's image: the therapist gathers the client's pieces and gives them back as wholeness (see Chapter 4).

Miller (1986) elaborates the phases of therapy for the narcissistic client who has encountered the depression under the grandiose defence. She details the process he or she can expect to go through: giving up on having old needs met; mourning and facing the pain of what you didn't get; feeling the full range of unacceptable feelings, and learning to ignore the demand to follow duty and instead begin to express impulses. She has a warning for the therapist that should be written three-foot high in the therapy room: *Never manipulate the client*, as this only strengthens the false self because the patient is so compliant. This is why CBT is a retrogressive treatment for depression: the client learns to self-manipulate, discredit their authentic feelings, and thus fails to find out why they are reacting to life with depression. The more the client comes from an external locus of evaluation, the more toxic is any kind of dismissal of his feelings as "irrational", because he will be further distanced from his own reality.

An existential view of depression can be useful in understanding how our world view can make us vulnerable. Existential therapy suggests that, like the psychodynamic concept of false self, depression arises in the gap between who the person is and who they believe they ought to be (Frankl), or in Boss's terms: they deny themselves for fear of losing the esteem of others (Arnold-Baker, 2005). Rogers (1967) understood the trajectory of therapy as the movement away from such an external locus of evaluation to an internal one, and this is the only way in which depression and anxiety will be ameliorated. In the depressed person the perception of the world is very narrow and closed, spatially, temporally, and relationally. He or she is frozen in a meaningless present with the past blocked off by guilt and the future by fear (Arnold-Baker, 2005). Exploring his or her guilt, fear, and belief system helps the individual understand the reason for the depression. Cognitive tricks won't alter anything if depression isn't used as an opportunity to understand one's world view and where it comes from, to engage with the childhood reasons for the shame, guilt, and fear, and to take the risk of moving towards an internal locus of self-esteem.

For individuals whose lives have been devoted to healing their depressed mother, taking responsibility for her happiness, and making reparation for her pain, what the client needs in therapy is to find herself. If she projects maternal neediness onto the therapist, it is crucial that the therapist conveys to her that she doesn't have to be good, compliant, competent, or efficient, that she can make mistakes and go at her own pace (Winnicott, 1984). The question for the client is as baldly confronting as "her own life or mother's?" (ibid., p. 94). For such a client the effort to wrest her own life back from her mother will stir up a well of guilt, and the goal of therapy is to lay aside that guilt. Feeling resentment against mother for the theft of her child's (the client's) life is a first step in therapy, but this will inevitably provoke more guilt. Susan has gone through these stages. She has placed some behavioural boundaries between herself and mother—she still lives on the same road, but no longer goes to see her every day. She has even generated some internal emotional boundaries—the guilt, remorse, and pain for her mother's loneliness and emptiness have diminished. When she was no longer in crisis with respect to her mother, Susan wanted to finish therapy with me, being terrified of having "nothing to bring" to the sessions. But her life was still unliveable: she was exhausted, depressed, depleted by friendships and social engagement, unable to return to work, and unwilling to commit to the boyfriend who competed with her mother for her attention. Yet she maintained that she was ready to leave therapy. Now I had become the demanding mother, and she, once again, the never good enough child. With Susan, my job was to provide holding and offer the mirroring she needed for the long task of finding her self and learning to create space for herself in relationships.

The somatic realm: the polyvagal theory

It should have become clear by now that the ideal therapist working with depressed and anxious clients needs to be knowledgeable and sensitive about developmental deficits, and to be willing and able to attune to and empathically mirror the client. No less important is the capacity to work with the emotions and body as much as the rational mind.

The polyvagal model (see Chapter 3) provides a neuroscientific grounding for what attachment-informed therapy has always known. It reminds us that the attachment relationship is embodied: recorded and expressed through the nervous system and other somatic processes. The theory also provides a framework for understanding which feelings (e.g. grief or anger) need to be felt and expressed (rather than repressed or denied); and which need to be heard and respected, but the situations giving rise to them not deliberately provoked (e.g. terror, or the response to threat in general). This is only possible in the context of a safe relationship, one that is mirroring, nourishing, and meaningful.

As we have seen, Porges proposes that safety is the treatment for trauma (2018). I would suggest that the same is true for depression: safety from the kinds of abuse, neglect, active or passive aggression, manipulation, misattunement, and boundary infringement that created the depression in the first place. If depression results from a prolonged state of threat to which the individual responds by cycling back and forth between the SNS and dorsal vagus, then resolving these threats is indeed the treatment. This requires cues of safety to be available: a soothing pitch and tone of voice, warm empathic facial expression. These cannot be faked on the part of the therapist, but must come from a genuine heart-to-heart connection.

Porges maintains that greater resilience to perceived danger and stress can be promoted by "neural exercises consisting of transitory disruptions and repairs of physiological state through social interactions employing cues of safety" (2018, p. 62). For example, for many people with an inflexible vagal brake, play can easily turn from fun into threat, as in the fear of humiliation. Therapy or other forms of warm, attuned contact can help the client become familiar with that border and learn to remain in a state of safety while playing. The aim of such work at the client's edge is to expand their "window of tolerance" between states of hyper- and hypo-arousal, and thus increase their self-regulatory capacities (Ogden et al., 2006). Down-regulating defensive states and facilitating states of calmness is achieved passively through the individual receiving relational cues of safety, and actively by the therapist helping the client to exercise the social engagement system in small increments (Porges, 2018).

Intentional appreciation of the present moment can be aided by mindful awareness of its different elements: thoughts, emotions, movements, body sensations, and the five perceptions (Ogden, 2018). This can be developed as a resource by oscillating between SNS or dorsal activation and the ventral state. The therapeutic dyad must identify which of the elements is easiest to activate and then think of a small challenge to exercise the vagal brake until the individual can easily move back and forth between unsafe memories and experiences of safety.

Therapists, even those who are generally empathic and attuned, do not always get it right, which provides an additional challenge and opportunity in the use of neural exercises. Indeed, even in healthy parent–child relationships there is accurate attunement only 30 per cent of the time (Dana, 2018), but the important thing is not so much perfect attunement as the willingness and capacity to notice and repair the rupture (Schore, 2003a, 2003b). When these ruptures happen between therapist and client, the response may be confrontation characteristic of activation of the SNS, or withdrawal, which signals triggering of the dorsal vagus (e.g. the client may suddenly be overwhelmed with exhaustion). But if the therapist notices and takes responsibility for the rupture, its repair can lead to a deepening of the therapeutic alliance, and the experience of ventral vagal safety and all that goes with this: a capacity for warm reciprocity, joy, exploration, and the beginnings of trust in relationships.

Everybody needs experiences of both solitude and connection, but the insecurely attached have difficulties with either closeness (avoidant type) or distance from others (ambivalent type). Both need to learn a non-anxious flexibility in moving between contact and separation. Dana (2018) has devised an exercise to practise this movement by savouring our independence as we breathe in and relishing our interconnectedness as we breathe out. During the exhalation, imagine the breath in synchrony with other people. Initially, the ambivalently attached will be challenged by experiencing separation as a place of loneliness, but by adjusting the length of the inhalation, they can learn to imagine it as a place of renewal. Conversely, the avoidantly attached may associate connection with judgement or invasiveness. They need to experiment with a continuum between wary proximity at one end of the spectrum and "joyful mingling" at the other end.

The vagus nerve bundle communicates in both directions between the body and brain: 80 per cent of its fibres (the sensory or afferent fibres) carry information from the body to the brain and 20 per cent (efferent) from the brain to the body. This suggests that therapy for dysregulation of the autonomic system (e.g. trauma, autism, depression, chronic anxiety) would be more effective if targeted at the body (bottom-up) rather than the brain (top-down): that is, body psychotherapies rather than mindfulness practices or classical psychoanalysis.

Bottom-up exercises

The vagus nerve can be stimulated via manual or electrical means, and left cervical vagus nerve stimulation is an approved therapy for treatment-resistant depression (Howland, 2014). This usually involves the surgical implantation of a pulse generator, but manual stimulation via neuro-fascial release can be done at home (devised by Rosenberg, 2017).

The ANS can be toned through sound, breath, or body exercises (all bottom-up approaches). Both the low frequency growls of predators and the high frequency screams of pain or panic signal danger, and it is in the middle range (such as the maternal voice) that we experience safety. A compilation of sounds (Safe and Sound Protocol) has been designed by Steve Porges (2018) to calm the ANS, and enhance resilience, increase sound tolerance, and assist with the screening out of background noise (a problem for autistic people in particular), all of which facilitates entering the social engagement system. Self-created sound such as humming or chanting "Omm" or singing in a choir enhance vagal tone and help to combat depression and anxiety. These exercises combine the benefits of sound, breath-control, rhythm, and relational reciprocity. Regulating breathing on its own also calms the ANS. In particular, deepening and slowing breathing down and lengthening the out-breath relative to the in-breath all enhance parasympathetic activity. Reducing airflow during exhalation (resistance breathing) is also beneficial (Dana, 2018). Sighing returns the body to a parasympathetic state, and indeed spontaneous sighs are a sign that various body exercises are working to that end. Dana notes how talking exercises the social engagement system through a variety of pathways (breath control, sound production, hearing, facial expression) and how conversation adds the experience of reciprocity as we take turns to speak and to listen.

Touch reduces depression, pain, and stress and elevates trust in the other (ibid.). A hand on the back behind the heart activates the ventral vagus, but if the therapist or client are uncomfortable with touch, an alternative is for the client to touch themselves over the heart or wherever feels comforting and for the therapist to mirror this. Social and physical warmth share common neurophysiological pathways, and physical warmth can be used to promote interpersonal approach (Dana, 2018). We can experiment with moving between social engagement and other ANS states by adopting different postures that express these states (ibid.).

When movement is inhibited, the processing of emotions is impaired because movement (including change of posture) changes autonomic tone—which raises questions about the usefulness of client and therapist remaining anchored in their chairs! For depressed clients, making the small adjustments to keep their seat on a therapy ball prevents dorsal vagus shutdown by engaging the vagal brake. Sitting upright in a chair is better than slumping because more positive events are remembered. A variety of movement exercises to stimulate the ventral vagus have been devised by Deb Dana and the body therapist, Stanley Rosenberg. For example, lying on the back with hands behind the head, look to the right by moving only the eyes. Wait until you swallow, yawn, or sigh, all signs of the relaxation of the ANS. Now repeat on the left (Rosenberg, 2017).

Effective help for depression comes from a variety of somatic approaches: exercise; exposure to sunlight and nature; a balanced diet, especially one rich in probiotics and omega-3 fatty acids; and treatment with acupuncture (Chan et al., 2015; MacPherson et al., 2013). These are discussed in more detail in my earlier book (Dowds, 2018) and won't be repeated here.

The emotional realm

We have seen that insecure attachment is characterised by dysregulation of affect, the avoidant individual tending to suppress emotions, the ambivalent to exaggerate them, and the disorganised to be the most dysregulated of all (Carroll, 2005; Dowds, 2014; Gerhardt, 2015). Knowledge of the cause of the depression is not sufficient to loosen its grip. Depression is characterised by the suppression or numbing of emotion, and it is essential to get the individual to recognise, accept, and express the emotion—usually sadness or anger—before they can move on (Lowen, 1973). Karla McLaren (2015) lived in a world where emotions were not allowed: sadness was labelled as weakness, anger was judged as loss of control, and the depressed person was shunned. She had no way of expressing her feelings about being abused as a child so she repressed them, thus becoming depressed—and then she had to hide the depression as well. Turning towards her depression and feeling the anger trapped beneath it saved her life and began the process of repair.

In 1820, long before Freud conceptualised depression as repressed anger, a London doctor reported curing a patient by provoking his anger (Coyne, 1985). The depressed man followed his physician's advice to see a famous specialist in Scotland. After taking the long journey he discovered that the expert didn't exist—but he was so furious with the doctor's trickery that his depression lifted. This recalls Fritz Perls' famous provocation: "Who are you depressed at?" Coyne describes an effective depression treatment programme where anger is elicited by continual firm but non-ridiculing criticism of the patient's performance of a dull task. When the patient blows up he is given social approval and assigned to a more interesting task. There is a health warning, however, in taking an anger treatment out of a therapeutic setting as other people become involved in anger and retribution and the feelings move beyond the control of the participants. There is also the problem that depression is often not primarily about blocked anger, but rather a response to trauma, to attachment wounds, and/or a failure of the self to develop. In these cases, blithely trying to raise energy through anger may fail, make things worse (e.g. by triggering anxiety), or hijack the more subtle and long-term work that needs to be done.

Anhedonia is a core symptom of major depression. Conversely, positive emotions are beneficial to mental and physical health, success and longevity, protect against stress, and predict a decrease in levels of chronic pain (Geschwind et al., 2009). Positive emotions can diminish the expression of genetic vulnerability to stress. Thus, boosting the ability to experience positive affect could play a role in developing resilience to depression, while the response to antidepressant medication may be conditional on restoring this capacity (Wichers et al., 2009). Barbara Fredrickson's "broaden-and-build" model hypothesises that the benefits of positive emotions stretch far beyond momentary good feelings: "A key proposition is that these positive emotions broaden an individual's thought-action repertoire: joy sparks the urge to play, interest sparks the urge to explore, contentment sparks the urge to savour and integrate, and love sparks a recurring cycle of each of these urges within safe, close relationships" (Fredrickson, 2004, p. 1367). In other words, there is a triggering of the primary emotions of SEEKING and PLAY that Panksepp (2010) has shown combat depression. For example, deep brain stimulation of the SEEKING system exerts powerful antidepressive effects in treatment-resistant patients (Coenen & Schlaepfer, 2012). One of the many ways in which reparative relationships assist in self formation is that they evoke love, which in turn elicits play and exploration. By contrast, a narrowed mindset is triggered by many negative emotions. The longer-term consequence of broadening momentary thought-action repertoires is the discovery of new creative actions, ideas, and social bonds. Siegel proposes that "inner positive states ... both arise from and support integration" (2012, p. 337). When integrated, "We accomplish more; we connect more; and we are more flexible, creative and adaptive" (ibid., p. 338). In other words, we experience a strong and resilient sense of self.

The experiential modalities such as Gestalt, psychodrama, and body psychotherapies are primary ways of experiencing and expressing emotion, and indeed, of playing and exploring. Body therapies include targeted (Weintraub, 2015) or exploratory (Grof, 1985) breathwork, working with the energy field (Chiasson, 2015), developmental movement (Frank, 2005), authentic movement (Hartley, 2005), or embodied-relational (Totton, 2005) approaches. They also incorporate therapies designed to work with trauma such as sensorimotor psychotherapy (Ogden et al., 2006) or somatic experiencing (Levine, 1997). Within these approaches we reconnect to our embodied emotional selves and also to the other in reciprocal intersubjectivity. Anxiety is characterised by restlessness, breathlessness, muscle contraction, vigilance, insomnia, chronic fatigue, or pain, and it becomes more irreversibly somatised the more it is ignored. Body psychotherapy approaches are essential to unlocking this somatisation, though acupuncture and deep massage may also be helpful.

Following the physical impulse (yelling, punching, choking, etc.) can facilitate the emergence of the unconscious process. In the words of Perls et al.: "If your orientation, your feelings and your actions come together spontaneously and with the proper timing, you will suddenly find that you understand, feel and can act with an unexpected new self-awareness and clarity; you will spontaneously recover a new memory, recognize what your true intention is in some present relationship, see clearly what is the next thing for you to do, and so on" (1972, p. 176).

Much embarrassment, fear, shame, and inhibition may need to be "worked through" before the client can utilise body approaches. However, if the therapist joins in and engages somatically him- or herself (for instance providing physical resistance for the client to push against) so that there is an overt psychosomatic relationship, such inhibitions begin to dissipate. This is particularly true if an exploratory, playful, and inter- active atmosphere is created, and indeed the play aspect of many body psychotherapy approaches and of psychodrama can be powerfully ther- apeutic in itself (see Panksepp above). Clients may learn to replace fear of novelty with curiosity, or may even learn to play with their challenges. Exploration in therapy relies on curiosity about the inner process, and once this is developed, challenging situations may even be welcomed as an opportunity for learning and developing confidence. Likewise, embarrassment at one's poor memory (or other perceived inadequacy) can be replaced by telling funny stories about getting into and out of hot water—how you managed to hide forgetting the name of the therapist you have been seeing weekly for three years.

Conclusions

To sum up, in working with a depressed client it is crucial to use an integrative approach, in which there is attention to the client's (and also the therapist's own) developmental and attachment issues, as well as to emotion, body sensations, and impulses, fantasies, embodied awareness of the relationship, and verbal expression. How some of these ways of working can be brought together in practice is illustrated by the case study in the next chapter.

CHAPTER 8

Brigid's story

Brigid comes from a rural working-class, conservative, and sexually repressive Catholic background, the oldest girl in a family of nine children. Her father was intermittently violent towards their mother when goaded beyond endurance (according to Brigid) and her mother passed the violence on by beating the children. She had clear favourites, with Brigid perceiving herself at the bottom of the pile. Mother withheld praise or affection from Brigid and treated her like a servant, even currying favour with neighbours by sending Brigid to clean their houses: "I was of less value to her than a sack of turnips." Brigid's mother had herself had a hard childhood, losing her own mother at an early age, being subjected to her father's alcohol-fuelled violence, and humiliated by illiteracy and class discrimination.

Brigid was able to move into the middle class through university education, working in IT and by marrying the local solicitor's son, who was now a successful businessman. By the time she came to see me, Brigid was in her mid-thirties and had a son and daughter. She was concerned about her relationship with her daughter, with whom she had never bonded—she said her daughter had been taken away from her by her mother and husband. Brigid was separated from her husband and they were in the midst of a legal battle over maintenance and access, and in the last year she had been forced to change jobs soon after taking out a mortgage on a house. She had been rejected by her husband during and after her pregnancies and felt bullied by him. She was consistently judged by her family (not earning enough; shouldn't have a mortgage; should be at home minding her children; being a "whore" for separating from her husband), who appeared to envy her education and apparent freedom. She was disturbed by vivid dreams of murdering people from which she woke with the most terrible guilt and anxiety, unable to shake off her sense that they were "real".

Brigid's day-to-day life was an exhausting cycle of chores (work, housework, children's homework, swimming, football, and Scouts) through which she dragged herself by force of will. Believing that if she ever gave herself a break the whole edifice would collapse, she kept going without mercy for herself. Her only visible emotion was resentment. She complained about bullying colleagues; about her abusive mother who she nevertheless depended on for childminding; and about her "lying, manipulative, self-pitying husband" who she was forced to deal with for the sake of her children. She always tried to do the right thing but was beginning to see that she was never rewarded for it. She believed she shouldn't manipulate her children about which parent they wanted to spend time with, but her husband apparently had no such qualms. When she complained about sexual harassment by a colleague she did so discreetly, yet her boss never trusted her again and forced her out of the company. Since her marriage breakdown, Brigid had gone on a few dates, but felt like a "slut" and was unable to relate freely to another man because of her sexual prohibitions.

Brigid presented in therapy as slim, attractive, and well-dressed in appearance, but she was jerky in her movements, with thin energy and a thin voice, eager to please and waiting to be told what to do. She displayed the characteristic symptoms of depression: poor self-esteem, low energy, insomnia, frequent sick days taken from work, low libido, a sense of emptiness about her successes, and a complete lack of joy or satisfaction in life. Having delivered an outline report of her childhood with almost no affect, she looked at me expectantly—as if I could now wave a magic wand and make it all go away. When, in a subsequent session, I asked where her feelings were, she said they were "trailing behind" her

(her mother had demanded a smiling face in public at all times against which Brigid was now rebelling). She had done some CBT before and didn't like all the homework, which was for her just a whole other set of chores to add to her duty-dominated schedule. When I said I was curious about which fairy tale would express her life myth, what she presented was a version of Sleeping Beauty that was really an amalgam with Cinderella—skivvy in the kitchen with envious stepsisters and a cruel stepmother, who poisoned her and put her to sleep from which she was waiting to be rescued by a handsome prince (or failing that, by me?).

I explained to her that, as part of our work, it would be necessary for her to feel the feelings, not just talk about them or try to get rid of them. In the court case Brigid went through great anguish, underlying which was a belief that good behaviour on her part would be met with justice: she was deeply upset at not getting *all* of what she wanted. Her pattern was to project blame and judgement onto others. However, using Gestalt chair work, she was able to get in touch with how *she* judged herself, and subsequently we worked on how she could develop boundaries against other people's judgements, demands, and perceived expectations. In one Gestalt embodied-boundary exercise, when I moved slowly towards her she initially stepped out of my way. With further challenge she put up her hands to stop me, but it took another major step for her to be willing to push against me. While she had a longing for freedom and the shedding of responsibility, I needed to help her to see that what kept her imprisoned were her own introjects.

Superficially, Brigid was an ideal client. She was able to get in touch with body sensations, easily came up with vivid images (shame as "sticky sludge", entrapment as a "straitjacket", etc.), and willingly worked with them. She had been employed in a company which presented itself as a cool and fun place to work but in reality treated its staff like slaves. To represent the straitjacket she experienced there she wrapped herself in a blanket and sat with her head down, unmoving and unprotesting. She came to the realisation that her entire life had groomed her for this, and she was then able to get in touch with self-compassion for having stayed too long in enslaving and bullying situations (job, marriage, etc.). She readily engaged in inner-child visualisations, made drawings and stories of herself in her family of origin—siblings all prodding her with spears—or of different conflicting parts of herself: for instance, thoughts, emotions, and body represented as flatmates who *had* to live together. All of this work was important and helped her to begin to *experience* the embodied affect which she normally held at arm's length.

Yet, as time went on, it became more and more apparent to me that while Brigid was doing apparently wonderful inner work, something felt missing. She was too passive in the absence of direction from me, and too compliant when I did make suggestions. Though her experiential work, images, drawing, and words all implied that she was in touch with her organismic experience, to me her affect seemed flattened. A number of times she said how happy she was with the work and thanked me on her children's behalf as well as her own. But I never felt that I was *receiving* anything on these occasions: no energetic transmission had taken place. Of course, flattened affect is part of depression, but what I really felt was that she wasn't in contact with me. I may have been the container but I was not a *person* to be related to. I tuned in to this by becoming aware of a gap, like a vacuum, in the space between us which her attempt at communication did not bridge. As a result, there was no real contact between us and our relating was static. Not showing her feelings might have been a dissociating or repressive defence, and/or a consequence of Brigid not experiencing herself as a subject at the centre of her own life. In other words, she had an empty, untenanted sense of self that generated the vacuum I experienced between us. Either way, she needed to learn that the affectless surface she presented had an impact on how other people responded to her. For example: a boyfriend ended their relationship without bothering to tell her; the judge in the court case accused her of lying, perhaps because she didn't show her desperation clearly enough to give herself credibility.

A breakthrough in *expressing* her feelings came when she finally trusted me and herself enough to play out an interaction between herself and her mother. Initially she played herself, and got in touch with her sense of abandonment, rejection, loneliness, and desolation at a time when work and her marriage were going wrong and her mother wouldn't meet her for a coffee or even respond to her request. At first she was reluctant to role-play her mother because of her fear of being or becoming like her, as well as her fear of being like her father and goaded into rage. I didn't pressurise her, and then she decided to give it a go.

In a first role-play she showed her mother's hurt, anger, and longings for her own life. In a second, her mother's hatred for Brigid as a child emerged: her loathing and envy of Brigid's prettiness, innocence, goodness, and intelligence and her being "loved by everyone". Brigid was shocked at the extent of the hatred and contempt that emerged in her portrayal of her mother, and I myself felt kicked in the stomach witnessing the violence of that hatred. This work helped Brigid start to: (a) realise that her experience was *true*; (b) understand where her mother was coming from, which made her responses less personal against Brigid and hence less destructive; (c) set a boundary around the hatred, which was revealed as coming from her *mother* rather than herself; (d) detach from her mother; (e) become aware of the impact of her mother on her expectations in other relationships; and (f) experience some energy, albeit here in the form of her mother's hatred. (A Kleinian analyst might argue that what this exercise displayed was Brigid's own hatred, but where would that hatred have come from if not from her mother? Indeed Brigid was well aware of her feelings of hatred towards her mother when she *began* therapy, so for her it was a shift towards health to grasp that she had almost certainly introjected that hatred from her mother. She felt less of a bad person as a result.)

A second breakthrough came later when the opportunity presented itself: it took the shape of *communicating* her feelings from a more subject-centred place of intent and agency. Brigid had unreasonable expectations of people in her life (husband, sisters, dates) and found it hard to put herself in their shoes or to negotiate with them. This later inevitably extended to me, which gave us a chance to begin changing her standard responses. Eighteen months into the work, she said that our current appointment time no longer suited her because she had to work late that night. She presented me with a single alternative. When I told her that I was not free at that time, she abruptly said she had to go to the toilet, something she had never done before in the midst of a session. When she returned—after some time—she switched into full "j'accuse" mode: "You are putting intolerable pressure on me … therapy is meant to provide support … I go to superhuman effort to get here every week … everyone wants something from me but I come here despite their demands … I pay you through the nose and the one time I ask for some flexibility you refuse." Then she started to cry.

Though taken aback by the onslaught and despite some quavering guilt feelings, I was immensely relieved that she had not simply walked away in silent fury, which I knew was Brigid's usual cut-off in the face of perceived rejection. I empathised with her life being so stressful and said that I wanted to support and facilitate her. We found that a Saturday morning would be possible for both of us in the short term and that her chosen evening would be free in six weeks' time (when some teaching was over for me).

This, I hope, gives some flavour of the work Brigid did towards taking charge of her life: inhabiting her self and becoming a subject at the centre of her own world. She started relating and communicating with others with more visible affect and better capacity to mentalize about her own and other people's inner states. As the therapy progressed, Brigid spontaneously became less driven by duty and began to go out with friends, express her creativity through painting, and explore a nascent spirituality and search for meaning—initially via tarot cards. She reported that her patience and empathic engagement with her children had improved and she eventually agreed to the children's father having joint custody. She stopped therapy after two years because of returning to college to train in interior design, with the intention of giving up her work in IT in favour of a vocation she felt passionate about. Her shame about having a sexual drive and her distrust of men as rejecting and sexually manipulative needed more work, to which I hope she will return.

Meta-commentary

I am aware that this description of Brigid replicates the flat way in which she presented herself: with little affect and as an object who was the butt of other people's subject-hood or egos. Experiencing herself as an object, she wanted me to fix her into being happy and feeling closer to her daughter. We didn't use the word "depression" during the work, and I believe it would not have been useful or enlightening. Brigid did display the symptoms of depression, but since she didn't use the D-word herself, I felt that using a pathologising term would have been a trap, since her deadness, poor self-esteem, difficulties in relationships, etc. were all *inevitable* consequences of her developmental and relational history and current life conditions. Within that context, her organismic and psychic responses were not at all pathological but, if anything, protective of the hitherto concealed but latterly emergent core self. Treating the symptoms of depression with antidepressants or with CBT exercises to combat negative thinking would have merely chipped away at the tip of what was an iceberg: a fragile sense of self shaped by poor relational experiences and manifesting as low self-esteem and, more significantly, as lack of subject-hood.

Brigid's attachment style was highly avoidant and distrustful, with some disorganised elements. Her mother was a narcissist, who couldn't see Brigid as an individual in her own right, as a subject, but did see her as a reflection of herself in the public world. Therefore, she was abusive towards Brigid in private, while boasting about her daughter's achievements in public, and indeed she could be violent towards people outside the family who threatened Brigid. Therefore, mother was a source of both threat and safety: the classic disorganising double-bind that leads to splitting off of the core self. Brigid had a strong will, which enabled her to achieve some superficial success in life, but it was a will oriented towards survival, and at the beginning of therapy there was almost no contact with any other organismic drives or impulses. She lived out of the vigilance of the sympathetic nervous system with regular dives into the dorsal vagus, such as at weekends when the children were with their father. She had neither a true self, nor one that was false in the sense of inauthentic; it was, more primitively, an adaptive self: one adapted towards survival. Brigid was not a subject at the centre of her own world: rather she was a collection of reactions to her own introjects and to the perceived demands of others. The intergenerational aspects of Brigid's depression are clear. Her mother's self-hatred, projected onto her daughter, arose from her own background of loss, violence, and alcoholism. Brigid's mother turned her self-hatred outwards, whereas Brigid turned hers inwards.

What influences triggered Brigid into feeling bad enough to seek help in the form of psychotherapy? A combination of elements played their part: stress and bullying at work, a job from which she was alienated and in which she felt trapped, the breakdown of her marriage, the adversarial nature of the court system, and the exhausting responsibilities of working full-time alongside bringing up two young children. With her keen sense of beauty, Brigid's surroundings were a continual offence to her spirit: the only place she could afford to live being an ugly, down-at-heel commuter town with few cultural resources, set amid flat, bleak agricultural land. There was no supportive community, no source of creative or spiritual nourishment, and no wider sense of connection, which might have provided meaning amid the day-to-day drudgery.

A symptom-oriented model would view Brigid's difficulties as a mood disorder. I have argued, however, that her depression is an understandable response to her early upbringing and current circumstances: her non-facilitating environment has generated and sustained a disorder of the *self*.

My way of working is experiential: rather than talking *about* how she felt, Brigid was brought into closer *contact with her feelings* through imagery, art, movement, and body sensations. This brings people out of the defensive, repressive dominance of the left hemisphere into the right hemisphere realm of embodied affect (Carroll, 2005). Working with Brigid's *relational patterns* took place in an implicit way: through my being warm, empathic, trustworthy, sensitive, and attuned—to the best of my ability. Research has shown that a high frequency of transference interpretations is detrimental to the outcome of therapy (references in Cooper, 2008), and my own experience is that clients feel embarrassed, threatened, or believe that I am blaming or complaining on the odd occasion where I have shifted from I-thou relating into a meta-commentary on what is happening between us. Allan Schore (2010) argues in persuasive detail that psychotherapy should rest on a relationship between the right hemispheres (implicit aspects) of the client and therapist, though of course the therapist's left hemisphere must be active too, but not in a dominating manner. While starting the therapy process being warm and empathic (two of Rogers' (1967) core relational conditions), it was essential for me not to go on indefinitely allowing myself to be "used" by Brigid. Just as the child moves from primary narcissism (mother adapting to child) to recognising the independent existence of mother and learning to adapt to her, so a client such as Brigid needed to learn to recognise me as a separate subject in the relationship, not just a resource which she paid to make use of. The opportunity came, as often happens, when I could not meet her needs, and firmly but gently told her so. In this process, she learned to negotiate, rather than cut off in anger as was her wont, and we managed to repair the rupture between us.

Thus, she learned that there are alternatives to, in Buber's terms, I-it relating. This was facilitated by my expression of Rogers' third core condition of congruence, where I was authentic in my response, while at the same time retaining warm acceptance and empathy. (For an integration of Rogers' core conditions with intersubjectivity theory and Buber's thinking, see Mearns & Cooper, 2005.)

This may all seem a far cry from working with Brigid's depression, but without this work of building a relationship and strengthening her self, Brigid would eternally retain an underlying depression even if her environmental conditions were to improve.

Conclusions

For long-term recovery, depth psychotherapy is essential: in this case example the causes of the client's depression were explored and in part repaired, and the individual had the opportunity to experience her interiority and get in touch with the needs of her true self. In other cases, some preparatory work may be necessary to enable the client to engage with their inner process. First of all, extreme anxiety, despair, or suicidal affect may need to be blunted with medication, particularly if the individual has suffered previous episodes of depressive breakdown. Second, negative and rigid belief systems that can be associated with depression must be challenged in order to clear the way for engagement with the inner process. This includes the client becoming willing to take responsibility for his own recovery and learn the lesson of his depression. This and subsequent exploratory psychotherapy must be held in a warm, empathic, and congruent relationship that provides the sensitive attunement and mirroring that have often not been provided by the caregivers in childhood. At stage-appropriate times, the therapist can become more than a facilitating holding environment and reveal him- or herself as a separate subject in the room and available for more intersubjective contact. It is essential that the therapy moves beyond talking about feelings to providing opportunities for the client to experience, express, and communicate them. Depending on whether the immediate trigger for the depression was loss or stress, the client must engage with the work of mourning or with calming the overstimulated nervous system respectively.

The repair of the self that Brigid required cannot be achieved by frustration, analysing the transference, or CBT tricks. Indeed the work here should not be seen as transferential at all, in the sense that it is not a re-enactment of the past, but aims to provide the kind of good enough developmental conditions that Brigid did not receive in her childhood.

Final thoughts

Depression can be experienced as an inexorable slide into a deep pit or a narrow mineshaft that sucks you in. This is Rilke's tunnel where "everything has become close/ and everything close has turned to stone". In such a process we are ruled by our dorsal vagus and, because "the mind narrates what the nervous system knows" (Dana, 2018, p. 35), all we can hear are repeating stories of defeat, despair, sadness, anxiety, self-hatred, and hopelessness. If it is the case then that it is not our brains that guide our lives but rather our nervous systems, what hope is there for the individual suffering from depression?

T. S. Eliot warned in "East Coker" that we should give up on hope, "for hope would be hope for the wrong thing" (1940, p. 200). If the wrong thing here is the demands of the ego, hope is indeed dangerous as it sets us up for disappointment and despair. This is because, in anything that matters, we are not in charge. As I am writing this conclusion in June 2020, the Covid-19 pandemic continues to gather force in some parts of the world, while abating, no doubt temporarily, in Europe. Millions of people worldwide are beginning to emerge from lockdown, but have lost hope for a world safe from the virus, for recovery from illness or bereavement, for a job in a time of economic collapse, or for ever enjoying the expansion of foreign travel again. So what can a depressed world or a depressed individual hope for in these times? Certainly, there are no guarantees, so to hope for specific outcomes would indeed be to hope for the wrong thing.

But what if instead we conceive of hope as "a basic orientation towards existence" (Pattison, 2015, p. 209), a sense of trust that life will carry us along, that some things will change and others won't, that our viewpoint is always limited, so that when we label an event or experience as "good" or "bad", we have no idea of the outcome in the medium and long term? So the challenge for the depressed person is to undertake the expansive spiritual work which leads her to trust that there are riches in her life, that there are days of light, that it is possible to answer the call of her depression by changing her contractive way of being in the world. As Eagleton has pointed out: "hope is performative", a self-fulfilling prophecy. It is far better to be hopeful as a basic orientation towards life because we will see the positive that is present even in the darkest times as well as the negative which will always also be there. And if the challenges become greater, we can allow hard times to teach us the treasures of life, the gifts of initiation, heart-opening, or soul expansion, the value of which is not instrumental but intrinsic. The stagnation of depression is the crucible that forges stillness and thus receptivity in the soul. This choice-less hope is not a "hope for ..." or a "hope that ...", which are the wishes of the ego. The prerequisite of such intransitive hope is, instead, "a radical abandonment of the [ego], a commitment to what one acknowledges to be beyond one's control and calculation" (Eagleton, 2015, p. 68). If we can learn to trust the wisdom of the Self, in the Jungian sense, we can let go of the survival-driven demands of the ego and accept and welcome what comes without clinging to specific outcomes. The stories we choose to tell ourselves matter. We should pay attention to the fact that the polyvagal and spiritual models we have described echo each other. They both emphasise the need to surrender the ego's dominance and illusion of control, and open to deeper sources of guidance. We can let ourselves be inspired by the redemptive hope of people who have transformed the suffering of depression into learning and initiation.

Glossary

Alleles:	alternative forms of a gene.
ANS:	autonomic nervous system, the part of the nervous system that controls the smooth muscle, cardiac muscle, and glands. Divided into the sympathetic (SNS) and parasympathetic (PNS) branches and mediates the fight-flight-freeze response.
BDI:	Beck Depression Inventory, a self-reporting questionnaire for estimating degrees of depression.
CBT:	cognitive behavioural therapy.
CNS:	central nervous system (brain and spinal cord).
Cortisol:	see HPA axis.
Cytokines:	molecules that help the body fight infection, but which promote inflammation when there is suboptimum regulation of the immune system. They induce one subtype of depression.

Default mode network: brain network active during waking rest that supports autobiographical memory, sense of self, and internal monologue.

EEA: environment of evolutionary adaptedness.

Endophenotype: a measure of gene function that increases the risk of psychopathology.

Epigenetics: the means whereby changes in the environment regulate gene expression through chemical modification of the gene.

Executive network: brain network that enables us to plan, focus attention, set and achieve goals. It must filter distractions, control impulses, and prioritise tasks.

GAD: generalised anxiety disorder.

Genome: the entire genetic material of a cell or organism.

Glucocorticoids: steroid hormones secreted by the adrenal cortex, of which the major one is cortisol.

Gut microbiota: the collective term for the bacterial species and other microorganisms that inhabit the gut.

GWAS: genome-wide association studies.

Heritability: the proportion of variance in a trait (reflecting differences among individuals) due to genetic differences in a particular population. The remainder of the variation can be accounted for by environmental differences.

Hormones: circulating chemicals produced in the glands which travel in body fluids and coordinate physiological responses by interacting with target cells.

HPA axis:	hypothalamic–pituitary–adrenal axis, one of the two major stress response pathways along with the fight-flight-freeze response of the ANS. The end product of the HPA cascade is the stress hormone, cortisol.
HRV:	heart rate variability controlled by the vagal brake.
Interoception:	sense of the physiological state of the body.
MDD:	major depressive disorder.
Mentalizing:	the capacity to empathically read and understand our own and other people's mental states and processes (e.g. desires, needs, feelings, beliefs and reasons) with some accuracy and sensitivity.
Myelin:	insulating layer around nerve fibres which increases the speed of conduction of nerve impulses.
Neuroception:	term invented by Porges for a neural process distinct from sensory perception which distinguishes safety from danger.
Neurotransmitter:	chemical which transmits a nerve impulse across the synapse (junction) between adjacent neurons.
OCD:	obsessive compulsive disorder.
OCEAN:	five-factor model of personality which measures openness (to experience), conscientiousness, extraversion, agreeableness, and neuroticism.
Pleiotropy:	the ability of a single gene to have multiple effects.

PNS:	parasympathetic nervous system, branch of ANS that enhances body activities that gain and conserve energy such as digestion and reduced heart rate.
Polymorphism:	a locus (site on DNA) with two or more variations in DNA sequence.
PTSD:	post-traumatic stress disorder.
Salience network:	brain network that detects and filters changes in the internal or external environment. The resulting emotional information mobilises adaptive responses.
SNS:	sympathetic nervous system, arousal branch of the ANS that increases energy expenditure and prepares the body for action.
TOF:	threat to overall fitness, an evolutionary model of depression.
Vagal brake:	the means whereby the ventral vagus regulates HRV.
Vagus nerve:	the tenth cranial nerve (really a nerve bundle) which regulates the PNS.

References

Alloy, L., Abramson, L., Smith, J., Gibb, B., & Neeren, A. (2006). Role of parenting and maltreatment histories in unipolar and bipolar mood disorders: mediation by cognitive vulnerability to depression. *Clinical Child and Family Psychology Review*, 9: 23–64.

Almaas, A. (2001). *The Point of Existence: Transformations of Narcissism in Self-Realization*. Boston, MA: Shambhala.

American Psychiatric Association (2013). *Diagnostic and Statistical Manual of Mental Disorders (DSM-5)* (5th edn). Washington, DC: American Psychiatric Association.

Arnold-Baker, C. (2005). Depression and apathy. In: E. van Deurzen & C. Arnold-Baker (Eds.), *Existential Perspectives on Human Issues: A Handbook of Therapeutic Practice* (pp. 189–196). Basingstoke, UK: Palgrave Macmillan.

Asay, T., & Lambert, M. (1999). The empirical case for the common factors in therapy: quantitative findings. In: M. Hubble, B. Duncan, & S. Miller (Eds.), *The Heart and Soul of Change: What Works in Therapy* (pp. 33–55). Washington, DC: American Psychological Association.

Badenoch, B. (2018). Safety is the treatment. In: S. Porges & D. Dana (Eds.), *Clinical Applications of the Polyvagal Theory: The Emergence of Polyvagal-Informed Therapies* (pp. 73–88). New York: W. W. Norton.

Barlow, D., Farshione, T., Fairholme, C., Ellard, K., Boisseau, C., Allen, L., & Ehrenreich-May, J. (2011). *Unified Protocol for Transdiagnostic Treatment of Emotional Disorders*. New York: Oxford University Press.

Barlow, D., Sauer-Zavala, C., Bullis, J., & Ellard, K. (2014). The nature, diagnosis and treatment of neuroticism: back to the future. *Clinical Psychological Science, 2*: 344–365.

Beckwith, M. (2015). The gracious, existential companion. In: T. Simon (Ed.), *Darkness Before Dawn: Redefining the Journey through Depression* (pp. 69–75). Boulder, CO: Sounds True.

Beebe, B., Jaffe, J., & Lachmann, F. (2005). A dyadic systems view of communication. In: J. Auerbach, K. Levy, & C. Schaffer (Eds.), *Relatedness, Self-definition and Mental Representations* (pp. 23–42). New York: Routledge.

Blazer, D., & Hybels, C. (2014). Depression in later life: epidemiology, assessment, impact, and treatment. In: I. Gotlib & C. Hammen (Eds.), *Handbook of Depression* (3rd edn) (pp. 429–447). New York: Guilford.

Border, R., Johnson, E., Evans, L., Smolen, A., Berley, N., Sullivan, P., & Keller, M. (2019). No support for historical candidate gene or candidate gene-by-interaction hypotheses for major depression across multiple large samples. *American Journal of Psychiatry, 176*: 376–387.

Bowers, M., & Yehuda, R. (2016). Intergenerational transmission of stress in humans. *Neuropsychopharmacology, 41*: 232–244.

Bowlby, J. (1980). *Attachment and Loss, Volume 3: Loss, Sadness and Depression*. London: Tavistock.

Boyce, W. T. (2019). *The Orchid and the Dandelion: Why Some People Struggle and How All Can Thrive*. London: Bluebird.

Brampton, S. (2008). *Shoot the Damn Dog: A Memoir of Depression*. London: Bloomsbury.

Bromet, E., Andrade, L., Hwang, I., Sampson, N., Alonso, J., de Girolamo, G., de Graaf, R., Demyttenaere, K., Hu, C., Iwata, N., Karam, A. N., Kaur, J., Kostyuchenko, S., Lépine, J.-P., Levinson, D., Matschinger, H., Mora, M. E. M., Oakley Browne, M., Posada-Villa, J., Viana, M. C., Williams, D. R., & Kessler, R. C. (2011). Cross-national epidemiology of DSM-IV major depressive episode. *BMC Medicine, 9*: 90.

Brown, G., & Harris, T. (1978). *The Social Origins of Depression: A Study of Psychiatric Disorder in Women*. London: Tavistock.

Brown, R., Duck, J., & Jimmieson, N. (2014). E-mail in the workplace: the role of stress appraisals and normative response pressure in the relationship between e-mail stressors and employee strain. *International Journal of Stress Management, 21*: 325–347.

Brumariu, L., & Kearns, K. (2010). Parent–child attachment and internalising symptoms in childhood and adolescence: a review of empirical findings and future directions. *Development and Psychopathology, 22*: 177–203.

Burcusa, S., & Iacono, W. (2007). Risk for recurrence in depression. *Clinical Psychology Review, 27*: 959–985.

Campbell, J. (1949). *Hero with a Thousand Faces*. Novato, CA: New World Library, 2008.

Carabotti, M., Scirocco, A., Maselli, M., & Severia, C. (2015). The gut-brain axis: interactions between enteric microbiota, central and enteric nervous systems. *Annals of Gastroenterology, 28*: 203–209.

Carroll, R. (2005). Neuroscience and the law of the self: the autonomic nervous system updated, re-mapped and in relationship. In: N. Totton (Ed.), *New Dimensions in Body Psychotherapy* (pp. 13–29). Maidenhead, UK: Open University Press.

Chan, Y.-Y., Lo, W.-Y., Yang, S.-N., Chen, Y.-H., & Lin, J.-G. (2015). The benefit of combined acupuncture and antidepressant medication for depression: a systematic review and meta-analysis. *Journal of Affective Disorders, 176*: 106–117.

Chiasson, A.-M. (2015). Practices to reconnect, retrieve, revivify. In: T. Simon (Ed.), *Darkness Before Dawn: Redefining the Journey through Depression* (pp. 99–112). Boulder, CO: Sounds True.

Cleland Woods, H., & Scott, H. (2016). Sleepy teens: social media use in adolescence is associated with poor sleep quality, anxiety, depression and low self-esteem. *Journal of Adolescence, 51*: 41–49.

Coenen, V., & Schlaepfer, T. (2012). Panksepp's SEEKING system concepts and their implications for the treatment of depression with deep-brain stimulation. *Neuropsychoanalysis, 14*: 43–45.

Compton, W., Conway, K., Stinson, F., & Grant, B. (2006). Changes in the prevalence of depression and comorbid substance abuse disorders in the United States between 1991–1992 and 2001–2002. *American Journal of Psychiatry, 163*: 2141–2147.

Cooper, A. (1986). Narcissism. In: A. Morrison (Ed.), *Essential Papers on Narcissism* (pp. 112–143). New York: New York University Press.

Cooper, M. (2008). *Essential Research Findings in Counselling and Psychotherapy: The Facts Are Friendly*. London: Sage.

Cortright, B. (1997). *Psychotherapy and Spirit*. Albany, NY: State University of New York Press.

Coyne, J. (1985). Towards an interactional description of depression. In: J. Coyne (Ed.), *Essential Papers on Depression* (pp. 311–330). New York: New York University Press.

Cozolino, L. (2010). *The Neuroscience of Psychotherapy: Healing the Social Brain*. New York: W. W. Norton.

Dana, D. (2018). *The Polyvagal Theory in Therapy: Engaging the Rhythm of Regulation*. New York: W. W. Norton.

Dash, S., Berk, M., & Jacka, F. (2015). The gut microbiome and diet in psychiatry: focus on depression. *Current Opinion in Psychiatry, 28*: 1–6.

Deurzen-Smith, E. van (1997). *Everyday Mysteries: Existential Dimensions of Psychotherapy*. London: Routledge.

Didion, J. (2006). *The Year of Magical Thinking*. London: Harper Perennial.

Di Pietro, J., Novak, M., Costigan, K., Atella, L., & Reusing, S. (2006). Maternal psychological stress during pregnancy in relation to child development aged 2. *Child Development, 77*: 573–578.

Dowds, B. (2014). *Beyond the Frustrated Self: Overcoming Avoidant Patterns and Opening to Life*. London: Karnac.

Dowds, B. (2016). Is life a bitch? The need to contextualise depression and realism. *Self and Society, 44*: 123–133.

Dowds, B. (2018). *Depression and the Erosion of the Self in Late Modernity: The Lesson of Icarus*. London: Routledge.

Dowds, B. (2021). Going beyond sucking stones: connection and emergent meaning in life and in therapy. In: R. Tweedy (Ed.), *The Divided Therapist: Hemispheric Difference and Contemporary Psychotherapy* (pp. 181–201). London: Routledge.

Eagleton, T. (2015). *Hope Without Optimism*. New Haven, CT: Yale University Press.

Eigen, M. (1993). *The Psychotic Core*. Northvale, NJ: Jason Aronson.

Eliot, T. S. (1940). East Coker. In: *Collected Poems 1909–1962*. London: Faber & Faber, 1963.

Eshun, S., & Gurung, R. (Eds.) (2009). *Culture and Mental Health: Sociocultural Influences, Theory and Practice*. Malden, MA: Wiley-Blackwell.

Essex, M., Klein, M., Cho, E., & Kalin, N. (2002). Maternal stress beginning in infancy may sensitise children to later stress exposure: effects on cortisol and behaviour. *Biological Psychiatry, 52*: 776–784.

Fisher, J. (2017). *Healing the Fragmented Selves of Trauma Survivors: Overcoming Internal Self-alienation*. New York: Routledge.

Fonagy, P., Rost, F., Carlyle, J.-A., McPherson, S., Thomas, R., Pasco Fearon, R. M., Goldberg, D., & Taylor, D. (2015). Pragmatic randomized controlled trial of long-term psychoanalytic psychotherapy for treatment-resistant depression: the Tavistock Adult Depression Study (TADS). *World Psychiatry, 14*: 312–321.

Foster, J., & Neufeld, K. (2013). Gut-brain axis: how the microbiome influences anxiety and depression. *Trends in Neurosciences, 36*: 305–312.

Frank, R. (2005). Developmental somatic psychotherapy: developmental processes embodied within the clinical moment. In: N. Totton (Ed.), *New Dimensions in Body Psychotherapy* (pp. 115–127). Maidenhead, UK: Open University Press.

Fredrickson, B. (2004). The broaden-and-build theory of positive emotion. *Philosophical Transactions of the Royal Society of London: Series B. Biological Sciences, 359*: 1367–1377.

Freud, S. (1917e). Mourning and melancholia. *S. E., 14*: 237–258. London: Vintage, 2001.

Fromm, E. (1990). *The Sane Society*. New York: Holt.

Frosh, S. (1991). *Identity Crisis: Modernity, Psychoanalysis and the Self*. London: Macmillan.

Garber, J., & Cole, D. (2010). Intergenerational transmission of depression: a launch and grow model of change across adolescence. *Development and Psychopathology, 22*: 819–830.

Gendlin, E. (1996). *Focusing-Oriented Psychotherapy*. New York: Guilford.

Gerhardt, S. (2011). *The Selfish Society: How We All Forgot to Love One Another and Made Money Instead*. London: Simon & Schuster.

Gerhardt, S. (2015). *Why Love Matters: How Affection Shapes a Baby's Brain* (2nd edn). Hove, UK: Routledge.

Geschwind, N., van Os, J., Peeters, F., & Wichers, M. (2009). The role of affective processing in vulnerability to and resilience against depression. In: C. Pariente, R. Nesse, D. Nutt, & L. Wolpert (Eds.), *Understanding Depression: A Translational Approach* (pp. 181–191). Oxford, UK: Oxford University Press.

Gibb, B. (2014) Depression in children. In: I. Gotlib & C. Hammen (Eds.), *Handbook of Depression* (3rd edn) (pp. 374–390). New York: Guilford.

Gilbert, P. (2007). *Psychotherapy and Counselling for Depression* (3rd edn). London: Sage.

Gnilka, P., Ashby, J., & Noble, C. (2013). Adaptive and maladaptive perfectionism as mediators of adult attachment styles and depression, hopelessness, and life satisfaction. *Journal of Counseling and Development, 91*: 78–86.

Gordon, J. (2015). A heroic passage. In: T. Simon (Ed.), *Darkness Before Dawn: Redefining the Journey through Depression* (pp. 11–24). Boulder, CO: Sounds True.

Grof, S. (1985). *Beyond the Brain: Birth, Death and Transcendence in Psychotherapy.* Albany, NY: State University of New York Press.

Guntrip, H. (1992). *Schizoid Phenomena, Object Relations and the Self.* London: Karnac.

Hackman, D., Betancourt, L., Brodsky, N., Kobrin, L., Hurt, H., & Farah, M. (2013). Selective impact of early parental responsivity on adolescent stress reactivity. *PLoS One, 8*(3): e58250.

Haig, M. (2015). *Reasons to Stay Alive.* Edinburgh, UK: Canongate.

Hammen, C., Hazel, N., Brennan, P., & Najman, J. (2012). Intergenerational transmission and continuity of stress and depression: depressed women and their offspring in 20 years of follow-up. *Psychological Medicine, 42*: 931–942.

Hammen, C., & Shih, J. (2014). Depression and interpersonal processes. In: I. H. Gotlib & C. L. Hammen (Eds.), *Handbook of Depression* (3rd edn) (pp. 277–295). New York: Guilford.

Hammen, C., Shih, J., & Brennan, P. (2004). Intergenerational transmission of depression: test of an interpersonal stress model in a community sample. *Journal of Consulting and Clinical Psychology, 72*: 511–522.

Hammen, C., & Watkins, E. (2018). *Depression* (3rd edn). London: Routledge.

Harding, M. (2013). *Staring at Lakes: A Memoir of Love, Melancholy and Magical Thinking.* Dublin: Hachette Books Ireland.

Harold, G., Rice, F., Hay, D., Boivin, J., van den Bree, M., & Thapar, A. (2011). Familial transmission of depression and antisocial behaviour symptoms: disentangling the contribution of inherited and environmental factors and testing the mediating role of parenting. *Psychological Medicine, 41*: 1175–1185.

Hartley, L. (2005). Embodying the sense of self: body-mind centering and authentic movement. In: N. Totton (Ed.), *New Dimensions in Body Psychotherapy* (pp. 128–141). Maidenhead, UK: Open University Press.

Hilt, L., & Nolen-Hoeksema, S. (2014). Gender differences in depression. In: I. H. Gotlib & C. L. Hammen (Eds.), *Handbook of Depression* (3rd edn) (pp. 355–373). New York: Guilford.

Howard, D., Adams, M., Clarke, T., Hafferty, J., Gibson, J., Shirali, M., Coleman, J., Hagenaars, S. P., Ward, J., Wigmore, E. M., Alloza, C., Shen, X., Barbu, M. C., Xu, E. Y., Whalley, H. C., Marioni, R. E., Porteous, D. J.,

Davies, G., Deary, I. J., Hemani, G., Berger, K., Teismann, H., Rawal, R., Arolt, V., Baune, B. T., Dannlowski, U., Domschke, K., Tian, C., Hinds, D. A., 23andMe Research Team, Major Depression Disorder Working Group of the Psychiatric Genomics Consortium, Trzaskowski, M., Byrne, E. M., Ripke, S., Smith, D. J., Sullivan, P. F., Wray, N. R., Breen, G., Lewis, C. M., & McIntosh, A. M. (2019). Genome-wide meta-analysis of depression identifies 102 independent variants and highlights the importance of the prefrontal brain regions. *Nature Neuroscience, 22*: 343–352.

Howland, R. (2014). Vagus nerve stimulation. *Current Behavioral Neuroscience Reports, 1*: 64–73.

Ikeda, M., Hayashi, M., & Kamibeppu, K. (2014). The relationship between attachment style and postpartum depression. *Attachment & Human Development, 16*: 557–572.

James, O. (2008). *The Selfish Capitalist*. London: Vermilion.

Jamison, K. R. (1997). *An Unquiet Mind: A Memoir of Moods and Madness*. London: Picador.

Jang, K. (2005). *The Behavioral Genetics of Psychopathology: A Clinical Guide*. Mahwah, NJ: Lawrence Erlbaum.

Johnson, S. (2019). *Attachment Theory in Practice: Emotionally Focused Therapy (EFT) with Individuals, Couples, and Families*. New York: Guilford.

Jung, C. G. (1956). *Collected Works of C. G. Jung, Volume 5: Symbols of Transformation*. Princeton, NJ: Princeton University Press, 1976.

Jung, C. G. (1963). *Mysterium Coniunctionis*. Princeton, NJ: Princeton University Press.

Kasser, T. (2002). *The High Price of Materialism*. London: MIT Press.

Kearney, M. (1996). *Mortally Wounded: Stories of Soul Pain, Death and Healing*. Dublin: Marino.

Keedwell, P. (2008). *How Sadness Survived: The Evolutionary Basis of Depression*. Abingdon, UK: Radcliffe.

Keller, M., Neale, M., & Kendler, K. (2007). Association of different adverse life events with distinct patterns of depressive symptoms. *American Journal of Psychiatry, 164*: 1521–1529.

Kelly, J., Borre, Y., O'Brien, C., Patterson, E., El Aidy, S., Deane, J., Kennedy, P., Beers, S., Scott, K., Moloney, G., Hoban, A. E., Scott, L., Fitzgerald, P., Ross, P., Stanton, C., Clarke, G., Cryan, J. F., & Dinan, T. G. (2016). Transferring the blues: Depression-associated gut microbiota induces neurobehavioural changes in the rat. *Journal of Psychiatric Research, 82*: 109–118.

Kelly, R. (2014). *Black Rainbow: How Word Healed Me—My Journey Through Depression*. London: Yellow Kite.

Kendler, K., Aggen, S., & Neale, M. (2013). Evidence for multiple genetic factors underlying DSM-IV criteria for major depression. *JAMA Psychiatry*, *70*: 599–607.

Kendler, K., Gardner, C., & Prescott, C. (2002). Toward a comprehensive developmental model for major depression in women. *American Journal of Psychiatry*, *159*: 1133–1145.

Kendler, K., Gardner, C., & Prescott, C. (2006). Toward a comprehensive developmental model for major depression in men. *American Journal of Psychiatry*, *163*: 115–124.

Kessler, R., de Jonge, P., Shahly, V., van Loo, H., Wang, P., & Wilcox, M. (2014). Epidemiology of depression. In: I. H. Gotlib & C. L. Hammen (Eds.), *Handbook of Depression* (3rd edn) (pp. 7–24). New York: Guilford.

Kirsch, I., Deacon, B., Huedo-Medina, T., Scoboria, A., Moore, T., & Johnson, B. (2008). Initial severity and antidepressant benefits: a meta-analysis of data submitted to the Food and Drug Administration. *PLoS Medicine*, *5*(2): 260–268.

Kitanaka, J. (2011). *Depression in Japan: Psychiatric Cures for a Society in Distress*. Princeton, NJ: Princeton University Press.

Kleinman, A. (2004). Culture and depression. *New England Journal of Medicine*, *351*: 951–953.

Kohut, H., & Wolf, E. (1986). The disorders of the self and their treatment: an outline. In: A. Morrison (Ed.), *Essential Papers on Narcissism* (pp. 175–196). New York: New York University Press.

Leader, D. (2009). *The New Black: Mourning, Melancholia and Depression*. London: Penguin.

Leahy, R., Tirch, D., & Napolitano, L. (2011). *Emotion Regulation in Psychotherapy: A Practitioner's Guide*. New York: Guilford.

Lee, W., Wadsworth, M., & Hotopf, M. (2006). The protective role of trait anxiety: a longitudinal cohort study. *Psychological Medicine*, *36*: 345–351.

Lessem, P. (2005). *Self Psychology: An Introduction*. Lanham, MD: Jason Aronson.

Leve, L., Kerr, D., Shaw, D., Ge, X., Neiderhiser, J., Reid, J., Saramella, L., Conger, R., & Reiss, D. (2010). Infant pathways to externalizing behaviour: evidence of genotype x environment interaction. *Child Development*, *81*: 340–356.

Levecque, K., & Van Rossem, R. (2015). Depression in Europe: does migrant integration have mental health payoffs? A cross-national comparison of 20 European countries. *Ethnicity and Health, 20*: 49–65.

Levine, P. (1997). *Waking the Tiger: Healing Trauma.* Berkeley, CA: North Atlantic.

Lewis, G. (2002). *Sunbathing in the Rain: A Cheerful Book about Depression.* London: Flamingo.

Lewis, M., & Ramsay, D. (1995). Stability and change in cortisol and behavioural response to stress during the first 18 months of life. *Developmental Psychobiology, 28*: 419–428.

Lin, L., Sidani, J., Shensa, A., Radovic, A., Miller, E., Colditz, J., Hoffman, B., Giles, L., & Primack, B. (2016). Association between social media use and depression among U.S. young adults. *Depression and Anxiety, 33*: 323–331.

Lowen, A. (1973). *Depression and the Body: The Biological Basis of Faith and Reality.* London: Pelican.

Luby, J., Gaffrey, M., Tillman, R., April, L., & Belden, A. (2014). Trajectories of preschool disorders to full DSM depression at school age and early adolescence: continuity of preschool depression. *American Journal of Psychiatry, 171*: 768–776.

Mabey, R. (2006). *Nature Cure.* London: Pimlico.

MacPherson, H., Richmond, S., Bland, M., Brealey, S., Gabe, R., Hopton, A., Keding, A., Lansdown, H., Perren, S., Sculpher, M., Spackman, E., Torgerson, D., & Watt, I. (2013). Acupuncture and counselling for depression in primary care: a randomised controlled trial. *PLoS Medicine, 10*(9): e1001518.

Madigan, S., Atkinson, L., Laurin, K., & Benoit, D. (2013). Attachment and interpersonalising behaviour in early childhood: a meta-analysis. *Developmental Psychology, 49*: 672–689.

Maletic, V., & Raison, C. (2017). *The New Mind–Body Science of Depression.* New York: W. W. Norton.

Marganska, A. (2013). Adult attachment, emotion dysregulation, and symptoms of depression and generalized anxiety disorder. *American Journal of Orthopsychiatry, 83*: 131–141.

Martin, L. (2008). *Woman on the Verge of a Nervous Breakdown.* London: John Murray.

Martin, L., Neighbors, H., & Griffith, D. (2013). The experience of symptoms of depression in men vs women. *JAMA Psychiatry, 70*: 1100–1106.

Maslow, A. (1943). A theory of human motivation. *Psychological Review*, *50*: 370–396.

McEvoy, M. (2011). *How the Light Gets In*. Dublin: Hachette Books Ireland.

McGilchrist, I. (2010). *The Master and His Emissary: The Divided Brain and the Making of the Western World*. New Haven, CT: Yale University Press.

McGowan, P., Sasaki, A., D'Alessio, A., Dymov, S., Labonté, B., Szyf, M., Tureki, G., & Meaney, M. (2009). Epigenetic regulation of the glucocorticoid receptor in human brain associates with childhood abuse. *Nature Neuroscience*, *12*: 342–348.

McLaren, K. (2015). Ingenious stagnation. In: T. Simon (Ed.), *Darkness Before Dawn: Redefining the Journey through Depression* (pp. 25–33). Boulder, CO: Sounds True.

Mearns, D., & Cooper, M. (2005). *Working at Relational Depth in Counselling and Psychotherapy*. London: Sage.

Mearns, D., & Thorne, B. (2000). *Person-Centred Therapy Today*. London: Sage.

Merkin, D. (2010, August 4). My life in therapy. *New York Times*.

Mikulincer, M., & Shaver, P. (2007). *Attachment in Adulthood: Structure, Dynamics, and Change*. New York: Guilford.

Mikulincer, M., & Shaver, P. (2013). An attachment perspective on psychopathology. *World Psychiatry*, *11*: 11–15.

Mikulincer, M., & Shaver, P. (2019). Attachment orientations and emotion regulation. *Current Opinion in Psychology*, *25*: 6–10.

Miller, A. (1986). Depression and grandiosity as related forms of narcissistic disturbances. In: A. Morrison (Ed.), *Essential Papers on Narcissism* (pp. 323–347). New York: New York University Press.

Mitchell, K. (2018a). http://wiringthebrain.com/2018/07/calibrating-scientific-skepticism-wider.html (accessed September 2019).

Mitchell, K. (2018b). *Innate—How the Wiring in Our Brains Shapes Who We Are*. Princeton, NJ: Princeton University Press.

Morrison, T. (2007). *Beloved*. London: Vintage Classics.

Murphy, K. (2020). *You're Not Listening: What You're Missing and Why It Matters*. London: Harvill Secker.

Nesse, R. (2009). Explaining depression: neuroscience is not enough, evolution is essential. In: C. Pariante, R. Nesse, D. Nutt, & L. Wolpert (Eds.), *Understanding Depression: A Translational Approach* (pp. 17–35). Oxford: Oxford University Press.

Nolan, P. (2012). *Therapist and Client: A Relational Approach to Psychotherapy*. Chichester, UK: Wiley-Blackwell.

Ogden, P. (2018). Polyvagal theory and sensorimotor psychotherapy. In: S. Porges & D. Dana (Eds.), *Clinical Applications of the Polyvagal Theory: The Emergence of Polyvagal-Informed Therapies* (pp. 34–49). New York: W. W. Norton.

Ogden, P., Minton, K., & Pain, C. (2006). *Trauma and the Body: A Sensorimotor Approach to Psychotherapy*. New York: W. W. Norton.

Panksepp, J. (2010). Affective neuroscience of the emotional brainmind: evolutionary perspectives and implications for understanding depression. *Dialogues in Clinical Neuroscience, 12*: 533–545.

Pattison, G. (2015). Death. In: N. Adams, G. Pattison, & G. Ward (Eds.), *The Oxford Handbook of Theology & Modern European Thought* (pp. 193–212). Oxford: Oxford University Press.

Pearmain, R. (2001). *The Heart of Listening: Attentional Qualities in Psychotherapy*. London: Continuum.

Pedulla, T. (2016). Depression: finding a way in, finding a way out. In: C. Germer, R. Siegel, & P. Fulton (Eds.), *Mindfulness and Psychotherapy* (2nd edn) (pp. 148–166). New York: Guilford.

Perls, F., Hefferline, R., & Goodman, P. (1972). *Gestalt Therapy: Excitement and Growth in the Human Personality*. London: Souvenir.

Plomin, R., DeFries, J., Knopik, V., & Neiderhiser, J. (2013). *Behavioral Genetics* (6th edn). New York: Worth.

Porges, S. (2003). Social engagement and attachment: A phylogenetic perspective. *Annals of the New York Academy of Sciences, 1008*: 31–47.

Porges, S. (2018). Polyvagal theory: a primer. In: S. Porges & D. Dana (Eds.), *Clinical Applications of the Polyvagal Theory: The Emergence of Polyvagal-Informed Therapies* (pp. 50–69). New York: W. W. Norton.

Porges, S., & Dana, D. (Eds.) (2018). *Clinical Applications of the Polyvagal Theory: The Emergence of Polyvagal-Informed Therapies*. New York: W. W. Norton.

Ravitz, P., Maunder, R., Hunter, J., Sthankiya, B., & Lancee, W. (2010). Adult attachment measures: a 25-year review. *Journal of Psychosomatic Research, 69*: 419–432.

Rice, F. (2010). Genetics of childhood and adolescent depression: insights into etiological heterogeneity and challenges for future genomics research. *Genome Medicine, 2*: 68–73.

Rice-Oxley, M. (2012). *Underneath the Lemon Tree: A Memoir of Depression and Recovery*. London: Little, Brown.

Roemer, L., & Orsillo, S. (2016). Anxiety: accepting what comes and doing what matters. In: C. Germer, R. Siegel, & P. Fulton (Eds.), *Mindfulness and Psychotherapy* (2nd edn) (pp. 167–183). New York: Guilford.

Rogers, C. (1967). *On Becoming a Person: A Therapist's View of Psychotherapy*. London: Constable.

Rolls, E. (2018). *The Brain, Emotion, and Depression*. Oxford: Oxford University Press.

Rosenberg, S. (2017). *Accessing the Healing Power of the Vagus Nerve: Self-Help Exercises for Anxiety, Depression, Trauma, and Autism*. Berkeley, CA: North Atlantic.

Roth, T., & Sweatt, J. D. (2011). Annual research review: epigenetic mechanisms and environmental shaping of the brain during sensitive periods of development. *Journal of Child Psychology and Psychiatry, 52*: 398–408.

Rottenberg, J. (2014). *The Depths: The Evolutionary Origins of the Depression Epidemic*. New York: Basic Books.

Rowan, J. (1990). *Subpersonalities*. London: Routledge.

Rowe, D. (2003). *Depression: The Way Out of Your Prison* (3rd edn). Hove, UK: Brunner-Routledge.

Rowson, J., & McGilchrist, I. (2017). Divided brain, divided world. In: R. Tweedy (Ed.), *The Political Self: Understanding the Social Context for Mental Illness* (pp. 87–113). London: Karnac.

Rudolph, K., & Flynn, M. (2014). Depression in adolescents. In: I. H. Gotlib & C. L. Hammen (Eds.), *Handbook of Depression* (3rd edn) (pp. 391–409). New York: Guilford.

Rush, A. J., Trivedi, M. H., Wisniewski, S. R., Nierenberg, A. A., Stewart, J. W., Warden, D., Niederehe, G., Thase, M. E., Lavori, P. W., Lebowitz, B. D., McGrath, P. J., Rosenbaum, J. F., Sackeim, H. A., Kupfer, D. J., Luther, J., & Fava, M. (2006). Acute and longer-term outcomes in depressed outpatients requiring one or several treatment steps. A STAR*D report. *American Journal of Psychiatry, 163*: 1905–1917.

Schore, A. (1996). *Affect Regulation and the Origins of Self: The Neurobiology of Emotional Development*. Hillsdale, NJ: Lawrence Erlbaum.

Schore, A. (2003a). *Affect Regulation and the Repair of the Self*. New York: W. W. Norton.

Schore, A. (2003b). *Affect Dysregulation and Disorders of the Self*. New York: W. W. Norton.

Schore, A. (2010). The right brain implicit self: a central mechanism of the psychotherapy change process. In: J. Petrucelli (Ed.), *Knowing, Not-Knowing and Sort-of-Knowing: Psychoanalysis and the Experience of Uncertainty* (pp. 177–202). London: Karnac.

Schwartz, R. (2001). *Introduction to the Internal Family Systems Model*. Oak Park, IL: Trailhead.

Siegel, D. (2010). *The Mindful Therapist: A Clinician's Guide to Mindsight and Neural Integration*. New York: W. W. Norton.

Siegel, D. (2012). *The Developing Mind: How Relationships and the Brain Interact to Shape Who We Are* (2nd edn). New York: Guilford.

Silberg, J., Maes, H., & Eaves, L. (2010). Genetic and environmental influences on the transmission of parental depression to children's depression and conduct disturbance: an extended children of twins study. *Journal of Child Psychology and Psychiatry, 51*: 734–744.

Simon, T. (Ed.) (2015). *Darkness Before Dawn: Redefining the Journey through Depression*. Boulder, CO: Sounds True.

Slater, L. (1999). *Prozac Diary*. New York: Penguin.

Solms, M. (2012). Depression: a neuropsychoanalytic perspective. *International Forum of Psychoanalysis, 21*: 207–213.

Solms, M., & Panksepp, J. (2010). Why depression feels bad. In: E. Perry, D. Collerton, F. LeBeau, & H. Ashton (Eds.), *New Horizons in the Neuroscience of Consciousness* (pp. 169–178). Amsterdam, the Netherlands: John Benjamins.

Solomon, A. (2014). *The Noonday Demon: An Anatomy of Depression*. London: Vintage.

Stern, D. (2000). *The Interpersonal World of the Infant: A View from Psychoanalysis and Developmental Psychology*. New York: Basic Books.

Stevens, J. (1989). *Awareness: Exploring, Experimenting, Experiencing*. London: Eden Grove Editions.

Sweatt, J. D., Meaney, M., Nestler, E., & Akbarian, S. (Eds.) (2013). *Epigenetic Regulation in the Nervous System: Basic Mechanisms and Clinical Impact*. London: Elsevier.

Tamir, M., John, O., Srivastava, O., & Gross, J. (2007). Implicit theories of emotion: affective and social outcomes across a major life transition. *Journal of Personality and Social Psychology, 92*: 731–744.

Thompson, T. (1995). *The Beast: A Reckoning with Depression*. New York: G. P. Putnam's Sons.

Totton, N. (2005). Embodied-relational therapy. In: N. Totton (Ed.), *New Dimensions in Body Psychotherapy* (pp. 168–181). Maidenhead, UK: Open University Press.

Tronick, E., Als, H., Adamson, L., Wise, S., & Brazelton, T. (1978). The infant's response to entrapment between contradictory messages in face-to-face interaction. *Journal of the American Academy of Child and Adolescent Psychiatry, 17*: 1–13.

Tronick, E., & Beeghly, M. (2011). Infants' meaning-making and the development of mental health problems. *American Psychologist, 66*: 107–119.

Tully, E., Iacono, W., & McGue, M. (2008). An adoption study of parental depression as an environmental liability for adolescent depression and childhood disruptive disorder. *American Journal of Psychiatry, 165*: 1148–1154.

Twenge, J. (2014). *Generation Me: Why Today's Young Americans Are More Confident, Assertive, Entitled—and More Miserable than Ever Before.* New York: Atria.

Verhaeghe, P. (2008). A combination that has to fail: new patients, old therapists. *Eisteach, 8*(4): 4–8.

Verhaeghe, P. (2014). *What About Me? The Struggle for Identity in a Market-Based Society.* J. Hedley-Prôle (Trans.). Melbourne, Australia: Scribe.

Vogt, R. (2018). Trauma severity: parallels between SPIM 30 and polyvagal theory. In: S. Porges & D. Dana (Eds.), *Clinical Applications of the Polyvagal Theory: The Emergence of Polyvagal-Informed Therapies* (pp. 285–302). New York: W. W. Norton.

Warden, D., Rush, A., Trivedi, M., Fava, M., & Wisniewski, S. (2007). The STAR*D project results: a comprehensive review of findings. *Current Psychiatry Reports, 9*: 449–459.

Watt, D., & Panksepp, J. (2009). Depression: an evolutionarily conserved mechanism to terminate separation distress? A review of aminergic, peptidergic, and neural network perspectives. *Neuropsychoanalysis, 11*: 7–51.

Weich, S., Patterson, J., Shaw, R., & Stewart-Brown, S. (2009). Family relationships in childhood and common psychiatric disorders in later life: systematic review of prospective studies. *British Journal of Psychiatry, 194*: 392–398.

Weintraub, A. (2015). Lifting the armor with breathwork. In: T. Simon (Ed.), *Darkness Before Dawn: Redefining the Journey through Depression* (pp. 57–67). Boulder, CO: Sounds True.

Wichers, M., Barge-Schaapveld, D., Nicolson, N., Peeters, F., de Vries, M., Mengelers, R., & van Os, J. (2009). Reduced stress-sensitivity or increased reward experience: the psychological mechanism of response to antidepressant medication. *Neuropsychopharmacology, 34*: 923–931.

Wills, F. (2008). *Skills in Cognitive Behaviour Counselling & Psychotherapy.* London: Sage.

Winnicott, D. W. (1984). *Through Paediatrics to Psychoanalysis.* London: Karnac.

Winnicott, D. W. (1990). *The Maturational Processes and the Facilitating Environment*. London: Karnac.

Wolpert, L. (1999). *Malignant Sadness: The Anatomy of Depression*. London: Faber & Faber.

World Health Organization (1993). *The ICD-10 Classification of Mental and Behavioural Disorders: Diagnostic Criteria for Research*. Geneva, Switzerland: WHO.

World Health Organization (2017). *Depression and Other Common Mental Disorders: Global Health Estimates*. Geneva, Switzerland: WHO.

Wurtzel, E. (1996). *Prozac Nation: Young and Depressed in America*. London: Quartet.

Yehuda, R., Daskalakis, N., Bierer, L., Bader, H., Klengel, T., Holsboer, F., & Binder, E. (2016). Holocaust exposure induced intergenerational effects on FKBP5 methylation. *Biological Psychiatry, 80*: 372–380.

Yehuda, R., Engel, S., Brand, S., Seckl, J., Marcus, S., & Berkowitz, G. (2005). Transgenerational effects of posttraumatic stress disorder in babies of mothers exposed to the World Trade Centre attacks during pregnancy. *Journal of Clinical Endocrinology and Metabolism, 90*: 4115–4118.

Zuroff, D., & Blatt, S. (2006). The therapeutic relationship in the brief treatment of depression: contributions to clinical improvement and enhanced adaptive capacities. *Journal of Consulting and Clinical Psychology, 74*: 199–206.

Index